How Anyone Can Become
A Lean, Fat-Incinerating,
Anti-Aging Wellness Machine!

CHRiS,
TAke 5 To
FoRTiFy !

How Anyone Can Become A Lean, Fat-Incinerating, Anti-Aging Wellness Machine!

Fred "Fit Food Dude" Schafer

www.fitfooddude.com

Library of Congress Control Number: 2004099310
ISBN :   Hardcover   1-4134-7762-3
                    Softcover   1-4134-7761-5

To order additional copies of this book, contact:
Xlibris Corporation
1-888-795-4274
www.Xlibris.com
Orders@Xlibris.com
23638

CONTENTS

SECTION IV
Help Your Body Win!

SECTION V
Help Your Body Win . . . The Workout

SECTION VI
Food and Nutrition Made Simple and Sane

SECTION VII
*Get You're Head Together . . . .
Because You Can't Get Very Far With Out It!*

APPENDIX

This book is dedicated to my wonderful wife Robin and my three terrific kids; Justin, Jillian and Joey. I continue to be amazed at how blessed I am to have them in my life.

You Will Learn

The 12 True Reasons people are unfit, tired, unhealthy and overweight.

How infomercials, diet books, fitness fads, prescription drugs, weight loss companies, the "Healthcare" industry and even health food stores often steer you away from enjoying extraordinary fitness, health and wellness.

The "Missing Link" to greater health & why most people are "looking for lean in all the wrong places".

How "losing weight" can sometimes make you a smaller, yet fatter, sicker, and weaker person.

The most effective fitness formula on the planet that will deliver healthy & permanent results in the fastest, cheapest and safest method known.

Why almost everything you need to know about nutrition you can learn from babies, cave-people and mothers. Discover simple methods for enjoyable eating to become and stay extremely lean, fit & healthy.

How to develop unstoppable motivation, confidence and excitement about the opportunity to live, serve and thrive through a lifestyle of leanness, strength and endurance.

"When health is absent, wisdom cannot reveal itself, art cannot manifest itself, wealth becomes useless, and intelligence cannot be applied."

Herophilus 300 B.C.

CONSUMER WARNING!!

The Fit Food Dude has determined that the following information may be excellent for your health.
Possible Risks and Side Effects Include:

- Ⓨ Vastly improved overall health
- Ⓨ Reduction in excess body fat
- Ⓨ Higher energy/endurance
- Ⓨ Reduced heart disease risk
- Ⓨ Improved skin appearance
- Ⓨ Firmer, toned muscles/body
- Ⓨ Reduced risk/better management of diabetes
- Ⓨ Increased metabolic rate
- Ⓨ Fall/injury prevention
- Ⓨ Quicker healing/recovery from injury
- Ⓨ Better gastrointestinal mobility
- Ⓨ Better digestion
- Ⓨ Better hormone regulation
- Ⓨ Greater flexibility
- Ⓨ Reduction/avoidance of arthritis
- Ⓨ Reduction/avoidance premature disease— disability—death
- Ⓨ Increased strength and power
- Ⓨ Sleep better
- Ⓨ Reduce cancer risk, especially colon cancer
- Ⓨ Lower resting heart rate
- Ⓨ Better ability to deal with stress
- Ⓨ Reduce/avoid high blood pressure
- Ⓨ More enthusiasm/hope
- Ⓨ Reduce/avoid osteoporosis
- Ⓨ Higher confidence/self esteem
- Ⓨ Greater ability to recover from cancer
- Ⓨ Enhance sport performance
- Ⓨ Enhance work and play performance
- Ⓨ Overall more active life
- Ⓨ Age far more gracefully
- Ⓨ Improved overall attitude
- Ⓨ Better ability to fight depression
- Ⓨ Feel better and look better
- Ⓨ Dropping jaws—from those around you who may be astounded at what a difference this information has made in your life!!

Acknowledgements

Thanks to the people who have personally helped me in so many ways during the writing of this book and also over the many years of preparation in getting ready to write it.

To my gracious wife Robin, who has helped me to refine my words with her wisdom and guidance. She has patiently tolerated my long hours of dedication to this project, while encouraging me in the value of what I was doing.

To my three terrific kids, Justin, Jillian and Joey, who with their combination of creativity and sense of humor make being a dad a real pleasure and joy.

To my sister Jeanne, who gave me words of support that helped me to expand the vision for this book.

To Nancy Williams, who has been a godsend in completing this book. With her extraordinary talent and continually positive and optimistic attitude, she has helped me beyond words.

To Ray Van Diest, who not only helped to edit the book, but also was one of the first people to demonstrate belief that I could actually write a book that would benefit others.

To my mother-in-law, Donna Fabig, who appears in the book and has always been one of my cheerleaders.

To Barry and Simon Schuster, who helped me to get started in the speaking business and website development, which ultimately led to this book.

To my father, Fred E. Schafer, who taught me the value of hard work and a down to earth approach to living.

To my mother, Betty Schafer, who has always believed in me and the adventures I pursue.

The information in this book is intended only for healthy men and women. People with health problems should not follow the suggestions without a physician's approval. Before beginning any exercise or dietary program, always consult with your doctor.

Care has been taken to confirm the accuracy of information presented in this manual. The author, editors, and the publisher, however, cannot accept any responsibility for errors or omissions in this book, and make no warranty, express or implied, with respect to its contents.

Introduction

Wiped Out by Killer Couches!

"We either make ourselves miserable, or we make ourselves strong. The amount of work is the same"

Anonymous

"Health is wealth. Always be sure to eat right and take care of yourself. Circumstances will come and go in your life, but if you lose your health, then you are really in a pickle."

My Mom

As a curious youngster growing up in western Pennsylvania, my first great ambition in life was to be a scientist. The world around me was simply fascinating. Animals, plants, mountains, streams, and the solar system seemed miraculous and complex. Countless hours were spent outdoors exploring and discovering all that could be found about the different facets of God's natural creation. Nearly equal time was spent indoors reading and researching anything I could get my hands on to learn more about the intricacies of nature.

As a teenager in the early 70's, my focus began to change. While nature continued to be a passion, a discovery caught my attention. I discovered that I was "physiquely challenged". This was a big problem, as I was about 13 years old, and high school was on the horizon. It became painfully clear that I was not physically prepared for what I knew would be ahead. I simply was not well matched with most of my peers. First of all, I was sick more often than healthy. I was also very thin and poorly proportioned. To make matters worse, I felt pathetically weak, and was uncoordinated and embarrassingly slow. I hoped that this was just a phase. Perhaps I was just a little behind and that would soon grow out of this awkward stage. But time was short because ninth grade was fast approaching. In my hometown of Pittsburgh, Pennsylvania in the early 70's, ninth grade meant one thing . . . . football! Never mind that I had virtually no football talent, football was what any able-bodied high school male did in our town. I was in trouble. My lack of physical prowess began to erode my confidence and self-esteem. I had to make a choice . . . and fast. I could accept my situation as it was or try to do something to make things better. I decided drastic changes were in order and I grabbed the bull by the horns.

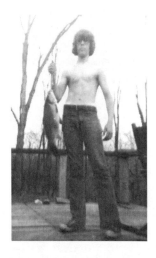

So with the same fervor that I had studied, researched and experimented with nature, I began to study fitness, strength and health. Throughout high school, I tried every form of exercise I could find. Simultaneously I foraged the fields of nutrition and bodybuilding to discover *anything* that could help me improve my physical condition, athletic ability, and self-confidence. By the time I reached my senior year in high school, I had achieved some success. I had put on about 50 pounds of healthy bodyweight. Although I never became an accomplished athlete, I was at least

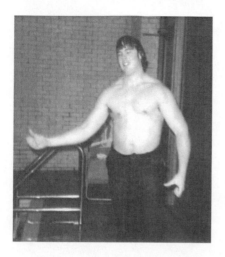

able to play high school football. To my surprise and delight, I was even able to go on and play small college football. I was enjoying the fruits of my determined efforts when another change came my way. In my second year of college, before football season began, I broke my leg. My activity level declined dramatically, but my food intake did not. As a result, my bodyweight shot up to 238 pounds, which in my case, was downright fat. Eventually, I needed to take that fat off. This new challenge proved to be a blessing in disguise, as it forced me to explore and conquer the intricacies and dynamics that lead to healthy fat loss.

As my new quest began, I began to experience a nagging, ongoing pain in my right hipbone and left shoulder. I went to several doctors and was quickly diagnosed with scoliosis, which is a lateral curvature of the spine. Apparently, I had possessed this condition for some time, and it was getting increasingly worse. My case was so bad, that one of the doctors wanted to use me as a "live specimen" to show his college students in anatomy class. The news was not encouraging. All the doctors told me there was little that could be done. This was in the late 70's, and the only solution offered was surgery. To make matters worse, I was told that the surgery was risky and may not fix the problem. With or without surgery, they all agreed that I would have difficulty bending over and picking up a pencil off the floor by the time I was fifty.

The only advice the doctors gave me was to back off on activities, especially weight lifting. I did as I was told and my pain continued to increase. After a few months of their remedy, I realized I hadn't noticed the condition to be a problem during the previous years of training for football. I also knew that I had nothing to lose, so I decided on a different approach. I aggressively increased my activity and weightlifting once again. The results were nothing short of amazing. I felt better and the pain began to dramatically diminish. I have continued to work out regularly since that time. The drawbacks associated with this 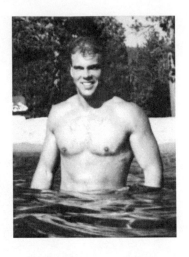 condition have, for the most part, been completely reversed and/ or contained because of ongoing exercise.

As I write this book, it is some 25 years later and Northern California is my home. In addition to still enjoying the great outdoors, my gusto towards a fitness lifestyle and the remarkable benefits it offers is stronger than ever. I have learned much about how to become superbly healthy and fit, and now have far more answers than questions. I have continued to be a fitness researcher; devouring anything I can delve into to discern one more nugget of wellness truth.

My findings have been applied to what I call a "healthiness lifestyle". As a result, as of this writing I am 45 years old, and in the best shape and condition of my life. I am able to accomplish many things physically now that I could not do when I was 18 years old. I've also been privileged to teach others the simple methods necessary to achieve their own optimum health and fitness through my personal training business and seminars.

For the past four years, I have traveled the country giving a speech entitled, "Life, Liberty and the Pursuit of Healthiness." As a result of this endeavor, I decided to write this book. You might ask, "Why did he write *yet another* book on exercise & nutrition? The bookstores are filled with them and the amount of information already seems overwhelming". The answer is clear-cut. One of my major motives for writing this book is that I have personally met thousands of people at my presentations from Fairbanks, Alaska to Fort Lauderdale, Florida who *have read all the books* but are still not enjoying extraordinary health. In addition, I meet people everyday in my community and through my work that say they desire dynamic healthiness, but are nonetheless puzzled as to exactly how to achieve it.

"Healthiness", by the way, is a term I use a little differently from others. To me it represents enjoying the highest potential of health, fitness, and wellness an individual can possibly achieve. This is not just the experience of absence of disease. It is enjoying extraordinarily good feelings of health and natural energy, coupled with a lean, fit and strong body that is capable of performing physical feats beyond expectation. I don't believe that this condition is the most important goal in life, but it certainly adds to quality of life, and makes daily living far more enjoyable and productive. I also know that it is possible for virtually anyone and does not require all that much time or have to be a complicated hassle. Unfortunately, the majority of people are still not experiencing the benefits of a "healthiness" lifestyle. Rather, most people sluggishly struggle along through the quagmire of mediocre or poor health and fitness.

This situation exists despite the plethora of instruction and resources available. Realistically, however, for those who truly desire to physically transform themselves, there exist few logical, effective, and complete solutions. I believe this is due to the following reasons. In life, regarding any subject, there is poor, average, good, better, and best standards. A great deal of the teaching available to the public, in my opinion, falls into the poor or average category. That is, it may help you to make some improvement, but not the kind that many are hoping to experience. The reason this situation exists is that most resources only provide half-truths or partial instruction.

That is, they may give some insights on eating better, but either neglect exercise altogether or give some vague reference to it. Likewise, many exercise books neglect specific nutritional guidelines or simply suggest following the USDA Food Guide Pyramid, which has not delivered optimum results in its current form.

Of those resources that attempt to address both food and exercise, little attention is generally given to the challenging "mental" issues that stop even the best-intentioned people in their health and fitness tracks. These mental roadblocks include becoming and staying motivated, being more confident in regards to health and fitness efforts, and then subduing the monster that we call stress. This dealing with "stress" issue is so vital because it saps much of the time and energy that we could be devoting to taking better care of ourselves and other productive endeavors.

Even worse than partial information on diet and exercise is instruction that borders on being non factual and untruthful. I am continually shocked by how little really good, sound and factual information is readily available to average, everyday Americans. Instead, we are constantly bombarded with gimmicks, less than the best methods and outright fraud. Unfortunately, these attempts to absorb your time, attention and money often come from the very professions that you are supposed to be able to be trust, such as fitness professionals and representatives of the medical field.

Sometimes this is not intentional. Instead, much of the time well-meaning professionals are giving advice based upon the limited or incorrect information they have accepted as sound knowledge. When it comes to the topic of healthiness, I ask the same question that news reporter Bill O'Reilly asks in the title of his book, "*Who's Looking Out for You?*" The answer, it would seem, is not many!

In fact, it often seems that no other field has more unsound practices, myths and outright deception than that of health and fitness. This condition exists for two principal reasons. First of course, is the almighty dollar. There is serious money to be made. By offering Americans the fast and easy "sitcom" solutions we are all used to, billions of dollars are being pocketed. Unfortunately, this situation leaves millions of people depleted of their valuable money, time and hope.

Second, the overwhelming majority of people do not understand the basic, scientific principles of extraordinary healthiness, especially with regard to above average fitness and nutrition. By the way, this includes many doctors and health care professionals. Doctors are usually dedicated individuals who have devoted their lives to improving the health of others. But with their burdensome schedules, most are not able to stay on top of the research regarding obtaining peak fitness levels. Most will tell you that "walking is the best exercise" and other vague information. While the advice they offer is not bad, it is only second-rate compared to what is possible for you. Certainly some doctors and other professionals are aware of better solutions, but they do not have a comprehensive and reliable source they can refer to with confidence. Patients are too often left in the dark to fend for themselves. This is about to change for you. In this book, I plan to tell you the complete, hard earned truth.

Point blank, for some of you, the information in these pages may save your life, if not extend it by 10-40 years. These statements apply to virtually everyone, despite their current age and condition. From pre-teenager to centenarians, anyone can improve, make noticeable if not miraculous physical, mental and even emotional progress, and have hope and enthusiasm for a brighter, fitter, stronger future. If you can move, you can improve.

A comprehensive, "tell it like it is" book like this is sorely needed. People everywhere tell me that they want a "system" of understanding health and fitness that will shoot straight, give simple direction, while providing motivation and encouragement. Prior to writing this book, I recommended other people's books, but not with full confidence. None, I felt, provided all that was needed to jump-start a lifestyle of explosively exciting healthiness. This book meets that requirement. Unlike some celebrities and talk show hosts who have decided to jump on the bandwagon, hire a ghostwriter, and cash in on the current obesity epidemic, this book is written from the *heart*.

A Fable for Our Times

If we do not turn the tide of increasingly poor health and fitness, I am convinced that thousands of years from now, when the history of our current culture is written, it will be titled, "Wiped Out by Killer Couches". As earlier mentioned, I really enjoyed learning about science and nature as a young child. Of particular interest to me at that time were the dinosaurs. Those great beasts that roamed the earth just astonished me. What especially fascinated me, however, was what had happened to them. That is, how and why did they become extinct? In those days, the reason that had the most credibility for their demise was the ice age. As I understood it, the ice age basically involved giant icebergs being formed at the North Pole. Then, due to their sheer weight, they began to slide south across the face of the earth, literally wiping out everything in their path. I remember envisioning huge icebergs descending across the face of North America, while dinosaurs looked up helplessly, anticipating their oncoming doom. It always puzzled me that they just didn't move. Now remember, I was merely a child. But it did not make sense to me that the dinosaurs did not try to escape. It seemed to me that they could have saved themselves by simply getting out of the way of the icebergs. Run towards the equator, climb up a mountain, something, anything to escape the giant icebergs! I used to think to myself, they could have saved themselves, *if they had just moved.*

Flash forward with me 2000 years from now. The scientists and archaeologists of that time will be studying our current culture in order to learn more about us. As they dig up the remains of our time period, everywhere they dig, they will find couches. They will be in shock and awe as they continue to find couches heaped upon couches. The interesting thing about these couches, however, will be the fact that most of them had indentations in them, apparently formed by human beings sitting on them for extended periods of time. And, in some cases, the couches had skeletons still attached to them. The researchers will be greatly puzzled by these discoveries, trying to figure out how these couches apparently overtook these people.

The first theory they came up with is that these were killer couches. Apparently they must have had some evil power, some ability to lull these people into lethargy, thereby causing them to sit themselves to death. But after further research, they will uncover information that will point in a different direction. They will discover that the couches themselves had no special power and they will realize that these were a people of superior intelligence. In fact, they will learn that they were the most technologically advanced people that ever inhabited the earth. Apparently, they will conclude, they developed so many technologies that they required less and less use of their bodies. These intelligent creatures finally reached the point of not requiring the use of their bodies for much more than what appeared to be their favorite activity and form of exercise, known as the "butt flop"—the activity of dropping down into these couches.

Researchers will discover that this phenomenon of consistent couch sitting began to slowly take its toll. Disease and illness began to increase. The humans of that time used their superior intelligence to develop medications to deal with the increasing illnesses. At first, the medications seemed to work, but as time went on, it became apparent that the medications created their own problems, and only made the people sicker.

In their increasing frustration, the people turned on the manufacturers of the couches, blaming them for the ongoing poor health plague that was sweeping across the land. Lawsuits began to be filed in great number against the couch makers, specifically citing the irresistible comfort of the couches as a major factor in creating the desire to sit for such long periods of time. The lawsuits were so great in number, though, that they got held up in court for years. Alas, it was too late. The control of the couches and the accompanying fitness famine of that time had taken its toll with a grip the people could not shake. Their intelligence and technological superiority had backfired on them and caused their eventual demise. Their knowledge was not enough. They gave into the lure of the comfortable couch and, in the end, were wiped out by a piece of furniture. As the scientists and archaeologists of the time conclude their research, they will perhaps wonder about this strange people who could have saved themselves—*if they had just moved.*

Now, I hope you realize that I am just having a little fun here. Sadly though, the picture I've painted is not too far from the truth. Inactivity and the resulting obesity it leads to are now the principal cause of poor health, premature disease and death in this country. On the other hand, purposeful activity—which is virtually free and available to everyone—is the most underutilized solution known for physical & health improvement.

This is a great country. It was founded, as you know, by tough, courageous, adventuresome people. Their purpose was to establish a place in which people could pursue life, liberty and happiness. Without great health, though, it is difficult to pursue anything. I sometimes wonder what the early pioneers would think if they could see our lifestyle. The emotionally overstressed, physically under stressed, couch potato existence we endure would likely baffle them. I believe it often baffles us. This brings us to a final question: Are you ready to "grab the bull by the horns" and begin the lifetime adventure of becoming a lean, fat-incinerating, anti-aging wellness machine? Consider your options for a moment if you must, and then let's get started!

The remainder of this book has been divided into seven sections. They are as follows:

Section One (Chapter 1) Overcoming Our Own Obstacles to Success: An in depth look at the Deceptive Dozen.

Section Two (Chapters 2-8) Abra Kadabra, Hocus Pocus . . . Give Me Your Money. How you can be hoodwinked into haphazard healthiness.

Section Three. (Chapters 9-10) Looking for Lean in All the Wrong Places. Why hope is possible for virtually anyone.

Section Four (Chapters 11-15)—Help Your Body Win! Exercise technology. Which delivers the greatest benefit, why you need it, how, where, and when you get it.

Section Five—(Chapter 16) Help Your Body Win . . . The Workout. Discover the most effective exercises on the planet!

Section Six (Chapters 17-19)—Thoroughbreds Don't Eat Twinkies. Food and Nutrition made simple and sane. Why all you need to succeed can be learned from babies, my mother, and those who lived off the fruited plain.

Section Seven (Chapter 20)—Get Your Head Together. Flexing the Muscle Between Your Ears, to pump up your motivation, enthusiasm and confidence while overcoming procrastination, self doubt, and fears.

Appendix—Additional resources for your continued healthiness.

Section I

Overcoming Our Obstacles to Success

Chapter 1

The Deceptive Dozen

The 12 True reasons people are unfit, unhealthy, tired and obese.

> *"Most people spend all of their lives developing one part of their body . . . their wishbone".*
>
> *Robert Frost*

Several years ago, a survey was conducted of Americans top priorities. In that survey, the #1 priority listed was maintaining good physical health. In fact, 97 people out of 100 listed this as their top priority. Maintaining a good appearance, less stress and the like followed closely behind. While you may or may not agree that these *should* be the top priorities of people, this is what they said. In reality, however, the survey also found that *actual* behavior is the exact opposite. According to the survey, only 3 of 100 Americans **actually practice** the 4 basic health habits of:

1)—Not smoking
2)—Maintaining a healthy bodyweight

3)—Eating a nutritious diet on a consistent basis
4)—Engaging in regular physical exercise as part of a lifestyle routine

Why is this? Were these people lying when they listed their priorities? Not likely. Rather, it appears that there are a myriad of reasons that people fail to make their health and fitness goals a reality in their lives. In this first chapter, we will look at twelve of those reasons. They are things we tell ourselves that can crush our quest for success. These are often incorrect, ineffective and negative thought patterns and attitudes that have held thousands, if not millions captive to a life of substandard healthiness.

This is one of the longer chapters in the book. It is feared that some may perceive it as a bit harsh. However, it is written from real life experience. Rather than shower you with sweet nothings, I have learned that those who seriously seek help can handle a little frankness in exchange for the possibility of greatness. I know that those who have helped me the most in life were those who were brutally honest with me in an attempt to help me be successful.

Statistics suggest most people who start reading a book never finish it. In fact, most only make it through three to five chapters. My ego would like me to think that this book will be different. I hope that you will not be able to put it down and that you will read it several times. Just in case that doesn't happen though, I have decided to "hit hard" in these first five chapters.

The intent of pointing out the negative is not to heap guilt or discourage in any way. Rather, it is to actually *encourage* you by showing that you are not alone. I want you to see that most people have these same thoughts. I believe that is why most are failing. They say half of winning any battle is knowing your true enemy. My guess is that you will see parts of yourself in at least one of the Deceptive Dozen; if so, you will now be better armed to defeat that deception in the future. If however, you are already extremely motivated and self-disciplined, you may think none of these "deceptions" apply to you. If that is the case, I invite you to read through them anyway. Perhaps you can encourage one of your teammates (loved ones or friends) down the road when they are faltering in their fitness endeavors. And lest you become discouraged, know in advance that the book concludes with a look at the life-transforming Delivering Dozen. Whatever you do, read the final chapter before you shelve this book.

Progression not perfection

One very crucial point must be made before we advance any further. My work is quite serious to me and I may sometimes seem intolerant of less than the best. At the same time, my sincere goal is your ultimate success. Success for each of us may look a little different, but it should be emphasized that everything in this book is based on "*PROGRESSION, NOT PERFECTION*". Brick houses are built one brick at a time, and that is how we are going to build our brighter and fitter futures! If a person were to attempt to get it all right at once, it would feel too overwhelming and lead to frustration and failure. Like a turtle runs a race or an ant eats an elephant, "one bite at a time," we will continually progress forward step by step towards better healthiness! So, without further delay, it is time to introduce the," Deceptive Dozen".

1) We Do Not Feel Worthy of Terrific Health and Fitness.

> *"Men go abroad to wonder at the height of mountains, at the huge waves of the sea, at the long courses of the rivers, at the vast compass of the ocean, at the circular motion of stars; and they pass by themselves without wondering."*
>
> Saint Augustine

We don't understand our real value. If it is true (and I think it is) that each person is created for a reason and a purpose, then it only makes sense to be in top condition in order to fulfill your destiny. Think about soldiers and competitive athletes. They train themselves in order to perform their best, often under demanding situations. And while we may not be in military battle or competing for an athletic championship, are our lives less important? If you see your life, mission, and dreams as not having significant value, you may have a tough time putting forth the effort to take care of yourself for the long haul. But think for a moment, if we are not of tremendous value, why were we all given different fingerprints? We are no accident, despite what some have been told, or perhaps have thought themselves. Each life is unique and each has a positive, purposeful and powerful calling. It is tremendously helpful to be in top condition if you hope to fulfill your destiny. Oh, and don't worry. Most of us will not need to train as hard as a soldier or competitive athlete. But we will need to train.

2) *We Have Become Physically Lazy, Undisciplined, and Unmotivated.*

> *"A little more sleep, a little more slumber, a little more folding*
> *of the hands to rest and poverty will overtake you like a thief*
> *in the night."*
>
> *Proverbs 6:10*

We all struggle from time to time with some aspect of motivation and discipline. But when it comes to a healthy lifestyle, it is critical that we don't let these negative attitudes/behaviors become habitual. If they do, they can create not only mediocre health, but also potentially life threatening, dangerously poor health. On the other hand, by overcoming these counterproductive traits, we can enjoy exclusively good health, a terrific appearance, and a higher degree of unbridled energy and enthusiasm for life. Whenever I feel lazy or sorry for myself as I approach my workout (or some other challenging task), I remind myself of how fortunate I really am. That is, I think of the thousands, if not millions of service men and women who have faced death or given all so that we might have the opportunity to live free and meaningful lives.

I also think of the thousands, if not millions of disabled people who would love to have the opportunity to exercise their arms, legs, and bodies. I imagine how excited those people might be to have the opportunities I presently have. This helps me to realize all I have to be grateful for and puts the discipline of exercising and eating correctly in its proper perspective. The good news is that *anyone* who is willing to put forth a *little consistent* effort can eventually have victory over these life squelching attitudes and behaviors.

3) We Have Given Up.

> *"A sad soul can kill you quicker than a germ"*
> *John Steinbeck*

I once heard Jack Canfield, co-author of *Chicken Soup for the Soul,* speak at a convention. He stated "80% of the population has resigned themselves to a life of mediocrity". They have simply given up. Nowhere is this potentially truer, than in fitness and health. One popular reason people quit is because they don't think there are really any viable solutions. Amidst the confusion and hype of the latest diet craze, people are disillusioned. If that describes you, keep reading! For others, this is not the case. Instead, they are simply exhausted. Life has worn them down, and they don't have motivation to get fit. Life has become overwhelming with demands of families, jobs and holding it all together.

What difference does it make anyway, they ask? Everyone else is in just as bad or worse shape than they are. While that is perhaps true, it seems a sad approach to take to life. We have a one-shot chance at living. Being fit contributes substantially to living an awesome life. And it's not all about us! Our attitudes, behavior and character will filtrate down to our children and be passed along for generations to come. When our children see us putting forth effort to take care of ourselves, they see that we still have dreams. That we are not done yet, and don't plan on quitting.

Most of us do not want to leave a legacy of lethargic living. Rather, given a choice, it seems most of us would want to embody and pass on the legacy of living life with an active attitude. Approach the opportunity for fitness and fully alive living with purpose, plans and optimism. As the poem "Don't Quit" says, "when care is pressing you down a bit, rest if you must, but don't you quit!"

4) We Want Instant Results.

"These are the days of overweight bodies and pills that do
everything from cheer, to quiet, to kill."
George Carlin

This is a bit of a double-edged sword. Part of the reason people fail to see and feel results quickly is that they are using ineffective methods. The truth is that there are a few credible programs that will produce *some* positive results if followed carefully. In that case, reasons people don't achieve their goals include not investing enough effort, modifying the program and perhaps most commonly, giving up too soon. They usually quit within a few weeks because they don't see the results they wanted fast enough. As we all know, we live in a microwave society and this impacts fitness as well. People want "drive up fitness" just like we want drive up food. Because most are focusing on the results they are seeing or not seeing in the mirror, they become discouraged when they haven't miraculously transformed within a few days or weeks.

This is a bit ludicrous of course, when one has usually spent years, if not decades getting themselves into less than ideal physical condition. I teach people "*Form Follows Function*". They feel and look the way they do because of the way they have lived their lives. Instead of focusing on looks, we need to train ourselves to focus on lifestyle and long-term health goals. I sincerely believe that the methods you will discover in this book are the best in existence. They will produce healthy results faster, safer, cheaper and permanently. I absolutely know this to be true and anyone can do it. *ANYONE.*

5) We Live As Emotional Junkies.

"If we only practiced when we felt like it, we would never have become champions".

Don Shula

It has been said that America is the most emotionally overstressed and **physically *under* stressed** society in history. So many people let emotions and feelings run their lives. And while emotions or feelings certainly have a place, using them as the barometer of our behavior often produces fluctuating (if not subzero) results. This is especially true in the physical realm. Putting forth physical effort is not something most of us "feel" like doing very much. But make no mistake, our bodies were designed for and need physical activity on a consistent basis. If our bodies are given consistent physical exercise and good nutritious fuel, they can stand up to most anything and be remarkably healthy. Most of us know this, but do not live this way. Often people will start off all gung-ho on their new and improved lifestyle system, and then a life stressor comes up. The first thing to go so they can "deal" with their stressor is their healthiness lifestyle. They stop exercising; start eating poorly, and loose sleep.

Usually, they continue on with the rest of their life as normal. They continue going to work, watching television, etc. Meanwhile the stress in their lives is building up in their body. It quickly leads to weight gain, sluggishness, depression, high blood pressure, slow metabolism, anxiety, diabetes, sleeplessness, digestive disorders, back and neck problems, heart disease, stroke and cancer. This is a lifelong habit pattern for so many, and it is a foolish way to live if you really think about it. We sacrifice our long-term health in order to handle present moment stressors. What is so important in your life that you cannot take 15-30 minutes a day to take care of your body?

Recently I read a study of successful centenarians. Centenarians are those who have lived to the 100-year mark or beyond. A "successful" centenarian is one who is still able to be independent or care for them selves most of the time. The #1 characteristic these individuals display has been described as hardiness. This term comes from the plant world and describes an ability to handle storms. The distinguishing factor of those with this trait is that they always take time to take care of themselves, no matter what is happening in their life at the time. This may sound selfish and self-centered, but these wise individuals have figured out that if they don't do this, they'll die. What good are they to themselves or anyone else if they aren't there? Let's follow their example. Our kids, spouses, boss, etc. will understand. If they care about us, they would prefer to see us happy, fit, healthy and productive.

6)   *We Live As If It's All or Nothing.*

> *"Don't let what you cannot do, prevent you from doing what*
> *you can."*
>
> John Wooden

In the book, *Think and Grow Rich*, it is explained that those who experience consistent success in their lives make big decisions quickly, and change them slowly. In contrast, those who live perpetually unsuccessful lives make big decisions slowly, and then change them quickly. There are many important, big decisions to be made in life. The decision to take care of ourselves would seem to be a "no-brainer". Yet, I have met many people with ample brains who are delaying or avoiding this crucial decision in their life. They seem to approach fitness as something that can wait, or that they can treat with an all or nothing approach. This is a sure-fire recipe for failure. Every year millions make New Years' resolutions to "get in shape" and every year, millions fail because of this "all or nothing" thinking. A certain sign of this behavior pattern are the words, "I'm waiting till . . .".

Rather than take this approach, I recommend that clients start training *immediately*, doing whatever they can. For example, if they do not have time for a 20-minute workout yet, start with a 10-minute workout and build towards a longer one. Or, if you have a bad back, do exercises around that area and strengthen the rest of your body until your back is healed. Check with your doctor first of course, but lets not kid our selves any longer. Remember, the goal is to make progress, not be a slave to perfection! Let me illustrate another way. Imagine that you bought a new plant. If you fail to water the plant regularly or if you choose to pour several gallons of water on it once a month, it would not thrive. It would probably die. However, if you give it a small amount of water and light each day, it will grow and stay strong and healthy. We are like plants. A healthiness lifestyle is our water and light.

7) *We Blame Our Parents.*

> *"I am never a failure until I begin blaming others"*
> Anonymous

Perhaps you are aware of a widely held medical theory that indicates we each have a unique genetic predisposition towards disease. For example, if your family has a history of heart disease, you are told that you are prone to heart attacks. What we have "inherited" though, is a lifestyle and perhaps a mindset that leads to greater likelihood of disease. I've thought this for a long time and have recently found several significant sources agree. According to the "The Nurses' Health Study: Twenty year Contribution to the Understanding of Health Among Women (1997) " . . . the contribution of genetics to most major chronic diseases remains small."

Allow me to explain further. Let's say you grew up in a home where perhaps your parent(s) smoked, had a few drinks in the evening, didn't exercise consistently, ate poorly, or had an anger problem (or all of the above!). Eventually, one of them had a heart attack in their fifties. Health professionals would tell you that you are at risk for a heart attack because of genetics. However, this may be true because of the lifestyle values you inherited and adopted, not because you inherited a heart condition. The huge problem with this myth is that people begin to view themselves as victims of their genetic make-up. They are lulled into thinking that their poor health is not their responsibility nor is it something they can change. A statement heard all too often is, "well, what can I expect . . . everyone in my family has had heart trouble". If you are not experiencing dynamic health, it is highly probable that you have been living an unhealthy lifestyle regardless of your genetics.

8) *We Are Appearance OBSESSED.*

We all want to look good. When it comes to healthiness, though, focusing on appearance as the *primary* measurement of success is a huge mistake. It is also a key motive for trying fad diets, stomach stapling, diet pills, etc. while practically ignoring true measurements of healthiness like body fat percentage, resting heart rate, muscular strength, etc. Focusing on appearance *first* is a reason many people never start or soon quit after starting a healthiness lifestyle. One woman at a recent conference challenged me with the statement, "O.K., lets say I follow your advice, how soon will I see results? Because if I don't *SEE* results right away, I'll quit". Based upon the number of people in our country who have never been able to stay with a fitness program, I think it is safe to say that this woman speaks for many. Here is the deal. **Focus** on building a healthier body and lifestyle first and appearance will take care of itself in due time. Great health and a good appearance really start inside, under the skin so to speak. The first and most vital goal is to improve our heart, lungs, arteries, veins, bones, joints, nerves and especially our muscular system. As we do this, our bodies will begin functioning as they should, and in a reasonably short amount of time, our outward appearance will improve. So many people feel like failures physically because they do not look like the super models or physique stars we see in the media. Because we can't ever see ourselves reaching such standards, some of us scrap the whole thing altogether. Remember, this is not about your looks.

This is about your life. Take care of yourself through a lifelong healthiness program.

As you do so, you will likely dramatically improve your appearance, possibly to a point you never thought achievable. But that will be an extra "benefit" of a better, wiser priority lifestyle, not as a result of a compulsive, neurotic, and all consuming fanaticism. Obsessing over body image has wreaked havoc on the lives of millions through eating disorders and low self-esteem. Appearance isn't everything. You should know that a recent survey found that people considered overweight individuals who exercised and were health conscious more attractive than "thin" people who did not exercise. The study showed that the exercisers were viewed as having a higher self worth, with more "pride of ownership" in themselves, and a happier, more positive, optimistic approach to living. Thus perceived as more pleasurable to spend time with.

9) We Have Made Effort a Four-Letter Word.

> "The human body was designed to walk forty miles a day and hunt saber-toothed tigers".
>
> Arnold Schwarzenegger

Measurements of efforts to resist stress have been measured on rats. Interestingly, the highest measurement of response and "aliveness" was when rats were put in the clutches of a metal hand that was slowly tightened around them. Initially, they showed little care and did not struggle. As the hand got tighter however, the rats began to fight back. Finally, as the rats perceived that death was imminent, their resistance literally went off the charts and the rats went berserk in their effort to live. The correlation I would like to draw is this. Why would we wait until our life is threatened to fight for it? Our society has painted a picture of an effortless life as something to be grasped. Even so called exercise books say things like, "Thousands of people are looking for some way to stay fit and healthy. They don't want to end up sweating, breathless and in pain". The author then goes on to describe how his program will meet the needs of those who view effort as an unnecessary evil. I am almost at a loss for words when I read something as nonsensical as that. Nevertheless, I will suggest that you consider three responses.

First, the ability to exert effort is what proves we are alive. When a person is no longer moving and their pulse is gone, they are dead. Why would we voluntarily head in that direction by progressively reducing the amount of physical exercise we get throughout our lives? Second, one of the best things a person can do for himself or herself is sweat. In fact, an ancient European health "secret" is to intentionally break a sweat everyday. This helps to cleanse and purge the body of impurities. When the sweat is brought on through physical effort, you get the added benefit of having life giving hormones released throughout your system. "Sweating the small stuff" daily is a wise practice and keeps the skin healthy too! Third, pain is not always a negative thing. For many years, the adage, "no pain, no gain" was popular. Now, many fitness and health gurus say that was all wrong. They would have you believe that you can achieve all your health and fitness goals in a sea of serenity and comfort. I say they are deluding us.

Look, no sane person really enjoys pain and discomfort. But let's define pain. There are two types of pain. Good pain and bad pain. Good pain makes things better and leads to more life. For example, as you follow the exercise guidelines in this book, you may experience a temporary discomfort in your muscles as they adapt to your new lifestyle. As you strengthen, stretch, and improve their condition, you will feel the "burn" that says your muscles are not used to this type of effort. This is *GOOD* pain. It means you are having an influence. Rather quickly, the health of your entire body and your ability to do some activities will skyrocket. This will require temporary, intelligently managed, small, progressive amounts of good pain. Bad pain does the opposite. Those who avoid all effort and feed their addiction to comfort, often end up with bad pain (such as diabetes, heart problems, cancer), and often, unfortunately, suffer for long periods of time. By avoiding GOOD pain, their bodies and health progressively deteriorate. They loose ability, strength, and vitality and experience increasing amounts of bad pain. Life without effort is an oxymoron. Learn to see effort as a good thing. Life is for the living.

10) *We Are In Denial of Our Substandard Healthiness*

> *"Who's afraid of the big bad wolf, the big bad wolf, the big bad wolf?"*
> Pig one and Pig 2 (Later eaten by the wolf)

A few weeks ago I walked into the office of a business associate and friend. He did not have the usual smile on his face and enthusiastic greeting. Instead, I could see that he was in misery and pain. His response to the customary, "How ya doing" was a grunt of agony. "What's wrong?" I queried. He responded, "My shoulder is killing me. I can't understand it. It never bothered me before. It came out of nowhere. It hurt so bad that I got a cortisone shot. I've got to do something. I can't go on with this pain".

Over the course of the past several years this associate and I have had several discussions on the topic of health and fitness. He continually makes jokes about his poor diet, lack of exercise and greater than average amount of excess body fat. At the same time he good-naturedly pokes fun about my dedication to a fitness lifestyle. Joking and humor is a good thing, of course. But I have had this same type of experience with thousands of people over the past twenty years and I have noticed something. When all of a sudden, "out of nowhere" they are diagnosed with a serious health ailment or worse yet, an LTD (life threatening disease), it is no longer a joking matter. There is not much humor when one must visit the hospital or must endure painful conditions and treatments.

There are no absolute guarantees in life. Like anyone else, I too could be diagnosed with cancer, a heart problem, etc. But the older I get, the more I realize how valuable the lesson of the "Three Little Pigs". As you may remember from the story, one pig built their house from straw, one from sticks, and the wise and diligent one from bricks. The pigs that built their houses from straw and bricks continually poked fun at Pig 3, as he worked while they played. Later, when the Wolf did arrive, the wolf destroyed the house of Pig 1 and 2. (In the original version of the story, they were eaten, but for the sake of children they were spared in later versions).

Here is the point. Many people continually rationalize that "I'm not in too bad of shape" and "I don't see the need for exercise or eating better". In reality, they are in denial. If they are not exercising regularly, they are not even *close* to being in as good a shape as they could be. And this applies even if you have a "physical" job such as a contractor, landscaper, day care worker, etc. While your job may be more physical than that of a desk job, it is still far below your physical fitness potential. And with the advent of technology and power tools, even our most physical jobs are not nearly as demanding as they were 30 years ago. Exercising, eating correctly and maintaining the proper attitude are the bricks to building a house that can stand against the ravages of time and the onslaught of stress. We can deny it all we want, but eventually, the wolf will show up at our door.

Poor health, diabetes, heart problems, cancer, bad backs and shoulders do not "come out of nowhere". Regrettably, like a plant that has gone without water too long, there may be no reversing the situation. Not much fun. More importantly, if you are not practicing a healthiness lifestyle, you are truly missing out on one of life's greatest pleasures. Feeling healthy and strong can cause you to feel like you could burst out of your skin most of the time and that is pretty awesome.

11) *We Tell Ourselves We Are Too Old and That It's Too Late For Us!!*

"Old age to me is always 15 years older than I am"
Bertrand Russell

"Most people die at forty, they're just not buried until they are seventy"
General Patton

Meet the greatest deceiver of all for those over the age of 50. Several years ago a potential client was discussing his less than ideal physical condition with me. He kept referring to his age as the reason for his condition. Due to the fact that he was only 13 years older than I was, I did not find his reasoning sound. I said to him, "So what you're telling me is that when I am your age, I can expect to be in the same miserable condition as you?" The thought of that seemed disheartening. Luckily, I knew better. Using advancing age as an excuse for poor health and fitness has been shown time and again to be unfounded. No doubt, advancing age has its effects on all of us and will ultimately take its toll. Still, most of us can enjoy an exceptional level of vitality and strength, even into our 90's.

Stories of inspirational seniors who run marathons, lift weights, climb mountains and deep-sea dive are becoming more and more commonplace. Dr William Evans, author of, *"Biomarkers: The 10 Keys to Prolonging Vitality"*, stated that "so much of what we call aging and its effects are nothing more than reduced activity levels, loss of muscle mass and an increase in body fat. By increasing activity levels, recapturing muscle and reducing excess body fat, we can greatly reduce the negative effects of premature aging and its associated chronic diseases." Eventually, the gentleman I spoke of earlier acknowledged that he had "let himself go" and has since been pursuing healthiness progressively and successfully.

Perhaps the ravages of poor health have already overtaken you. Maybe cancer, heart disease, diabetes or another chronic and serious health issue is current reality in your life. By employing the concepts suggested throughout this book, I am confident you can significantly improve your condition. Research projects using similar techniques to the ones I suggest have been conducted in nursing homes and cancer clinics where participants have been able to increase strength levels 110%, give up their wheelchairs and walkers, and regain independence and hope. Some of these participants were in their late 80's and 90's and most had one or more serious chronic diseases. You are not too old and it is not too late for you. If you can move, you can always improve! If you have not practiced a fitness lifestyle for some time, it may take you a little longer to "get back in the saddle". But every day you wait makes that saddle look a little more intimidating! Check with your doctor, show him this book, e-mail me if you need additional guidance. Do whatever it takes, but get started today!!

12) *We Don't Understand the Principles of Time or Energy.*

> *"Time waits for no one and it won't wait for me"*
> *The Rolling Stones*

How each of uses our time defines our life. We have all heard the adage, "each of us is given the same 24 hours, and it's how we use it that makes the difference". So many people I talk with state "lack of time" as a predominant reason for not pursuing their fitness goals. Sadly, these folks just don't understand how little time it will really take to dramatically improve their health. Granted, most everyone is busy. We all have demanding schedules. I find it interesting though that both Presidents Bush and Clinton made time EVERY DAY to exercise. In fact, George Bush has been tested and is ranked in the top 1% of men his age for fitness levels. Apparently, he understands how crucial health and fitness are to being at the top of his game. This will probably offend some of you, but I do not think there is anyone on the planet that is too busy to exercise. Instead, it is highly likely that you could improve your time management by removing a less productive activity. At the same time, you may not understand that exercise, health and fitness do not TAKE time, they MAKE time.

Recently I spoke with a Doctor who has implemented most of the concepts of this book into his life. He told me that he now gets up to two more hours of productivity out of his day, requires less sleep, and misses less work from illness and visits to the chiropractor. Thus, his healthiness lifestyle is *adding* time to his life! Even 15 minutes of good training can yield 2 hours of increased productivity to your day.

Several studies with corporate wellness programs provide overwhelming evidence of the time and cost savings that healthier and fit employees realize for themselves and their company. On the other hand, if you don't make time for healthiness, you'll have to make time to feel like crud. People who know this view a healthiness lifestyle as a wise investment in their future that pays for its self today and for decades to come. Let's break this whole time issue down and put it into perspective.

As you know, there are 24 hours in a day, which equals 168 hours in a week. Most people sleep 8 hours a day (or less). That leaves 112 waking hours in a week—or 6720 minutes. If you worked out 20 minutes a day, 7 days a week, you would spend a total of 140 minutes exercising. That amount of time is equal to only 2.08 % of your waking hours. Surely your life, health and future are worth investing 2.08 % of your time. You can even add further value to your fitness time by listening to books on tape or inspiring music. Did you know that being out of shape could reduce your life expectancy by 10-40 years? Being fit can ADD 10-40 years. Be smart—invest now.

In the last section of this book, I will share ideas on how to more effectively use your time and incorporate healthiness into a lifestyle "rhythm". Numerous individuals view healthiness as something that they must add to an already weary load. Instead, we will look at what can be "worked out" of your life as we progressively work healthiness in. In my work as a fitness trainer, I literally spend as much time as an "excuse eraser" and lifestyle coach as I do in actual fitness instruction. If this is an area of struggle for you, the good news is that you can potentially add decades of high quality time to your life.

And what about energy? Energy is a funny thing. The less you expend or invest of it, the less you will have. People often build up in their minds a false idea of how much energy a fitness lifestyle requires. But like everything taught in this book, you are encouraged to *progressively* increase your energy output. As a result, you will progressively gain energy. Interestingly enough, in many cases those who take up a healthiness lifestyle soon find themselves with so much more energy that they WANT to expend more energy! It is not uncommon for clients to take up activities they had given up as being "for younger people" after a few months of training. This much we know for sure. If the person who "has no energy" does not *force* himself or herself to start expending productive and healthy energy on a programmed basis, they will continue to see their productive and healthy energy levels insidiously slip—slide away.

Hopefully this chapter has made you more aware of how the "Deceptive Dozen" can operate as falsehoods, excuses and negative attitudes in your life. Though they may have drifted into your habitual thinking and shipwrecked your success in the past, perhaps you are now better prepared to avoid crashing into these icebergs of illusion that may have kept you frozen in your tracks. The goal is to get you to start and stay on a straighter course. Eventually that straighter course will include proactive action on your part! But alas, we are not out of dangerous waters yet. There are still treacherous trickeries waiting to torpedo our honorable pursuits of life, liberty and healthiness and keep us from reaching the shores of triumph. The difficulty with these trickeries and deceptions is that they are often masters of disguise. While they may appear as friendly rescuers able to save us, they are truly pirates of our healthiness treasure. Their one and only goal is to pillage our hard earned cash, plunder our hopes and then leave us as health and fitness cast-a-bouts.

In some cases these intended rescuers may be friendly and admirable in their intent. But, what they fail to tell you is that their own ship has leaks and is likely to sink. Although their ship may be a better choice than the pirates, they cannot save us either because they themselves have never been able to make it to the shoreline of abundant healthiness. Never fear, as we chart our way through chapters 2-8, we will see the fog of fraud lifting and begin to head into the horizon of authentic lifelong healthiness.

Section II

Abra Kadaba, Hocus Pocus . . .
Give Me Your Money!

Chapter 2

Fitness Fairy Tales and Fitness Frogs

As a teenager growing up in the 1970's, the comedians Cheech and Chong were very popular. Although they were not known for their contributions to the fields of health and wellness, they did leave us with an illustration of why so many are failing to reach their healthiness goals. The one thing that I remember most about Cheech and Chong was their version of, "The Night Before Christmas". At the end of the story, Cheech says to Chong, "Uh man, I gotta question. What was their secret? I mean like, Santa Claus and the little tiny reindeer. How did those dudes fly maaan?" Chong responds, "Oh man, that's no secret, everybody knows that man, they took the *MAGIC DUST*!"

You may be asking yourself, what the heck does that have to do with health and fitness? Well, I'm glad you asked. You see, rarely does a week go by that I do not hear a similar conversation in regards to the pursuit of greater health. Whether it is a personal conversation, television commercial, newspaper or radio advertisement, it seems that someone is always looking for or selling fitness magic dust. We are too easily fooled into thinking that there is a magic potion that we can take that we can take and "poof!"—we become instantly fit, healthy and well. Well, after nearly thirty years of research and application, there is one thing in this lifetime of which I am *ABSOLUTELY* certain. When it comes to our fitness, health and wellness, there is no magic dust. And while many of you may still be wanting to believe there is and are still searching for it, there are just as many out there willing to sell you their version of magic dust. What exactly do I mean by magic dust?

Magic dust is *anything* that tells you that you can get instant, amazing and miraculous results with no effort, no self-discipline and no change in lifestyle. Another term to describe this spectacle is "junk science". "Oh come on now, none of us would be so gullible as to fall for anything like that! We all know that something that looks too good to be true usually is!" Really? Did you know that approximately $55 *BILLION* dollars a year is spent on weight loss gimmicks that do not work? How can this be? In this section of the book we will examine several ways this happens to well intentioned Americans every day of the year, year after year.

Have you watched any late night or early Sunday morning T.V lately? If so, perhaps you have seen the healthiness horror show known as "the piece of junk fitness equipment that will swallow up your abs". Actually, it is not usually a show, but an advertisement that may go on for what seems like hours. Oh don't worry, if you missed the show you can see the latest episode the next time you go garage sale shopping. Because that is where these fitness-gizmo-fairytale-pieces of rubbish eventually find themselves. Now, I am not going to name any names but I would like to help you distinguish trash from truth. And this can be difficult. You see, there are now a few (very few) pieces of legitimate equipment being sold on television by trustworthy companies. Advertising on television though, by its nature, is meant to captivate and convince us to purchase. So, even these good companies have that element of "too good to be true glitz" about them. If they came out and told you the straight truth, it might sound like this, "the people demonstrating our equipment did not develop *most* of their fine physique using our equipment. Rather, they have spent at least five years consistently working hard, most likely lifting weights, running, calisthenics and being disciplined in their overall lifestyle including eating very well. You too can dramatically improve your health and appearance if you will adopt the same lifestyle, attitude and commitment that they have. Otherwise, you can purchase all the equipment you want, but unless you use it diligently (longer than three weeks) along with improving all related areas in your life, you will be simply wasting your money."

Obviously, that would not sell very well, albeit the truth. What makes matters even worse is that respected and once responsible fitness trainers are now in on the act. These are generally people who got started in their careers by teaching legitimate truths that could help people. As a result of their once positive efforts, some of them gained a great deal of notoriety and even have had their own television shows. But hey, telling the truth does not sell well. So, in my opinion, these once credible fitness trainers have given in to the temptation to cash in on a trusting and hopeful public. And cash in they have! A recent product advertised allowed you to sit on your derriere and lean forward or back while proposing to develop amazing abs. It sold well into the billions of dollars. I've heard that the promoter of this product defended its virtue. His argument was basically that people are going to spend their money on these types of products anyway. Therefore, we as trainers should develop and market products like this in order to "hook" potential clients and then teach them that a product like ours is only a small part of a fitness lifestyle. Collect your four monthly payments of $19.95 first, of course!

Another underlying problem with these products is that the people who purchase this stuff are usually not ready to commit to a true healthiness lifestyle. In fact, I have yet to meet *anyone* who has bought "cheap, fast and easy fitness equipment" who had the correct mindset to become healthier. Usually, they have conditioned themselves to believe that drive up fitness and microwave muscles really does exist. If you believe that, stay tuned because I am in the process of developing an incredible product that will make all your dreams come true! That's right, with my new, "Freddie the Fitness Frog, you will simply have to hold him in your hands, close your eyes, make your fitness wish, give him a kiss, and voila, you will be transformed into someone with amazing health. In as little as 3 seconds a day with only one easy payment of $19.95 . . . sound familiar? I bet it would sell. O.K., enough sarcasm.

I may never get rich telling people the candid fitness facts and healthiness truth. There is just no getting around the truth. Real healthiness will require you to do something and keep doing it over the long haul. Positive, proactive, productive action on our part is what makes good things happen. At the same time, I choose to believe the best about people and know in my heart of hearts that anyone can do what I'm suggesting. Real hope and encouragement along with facts that can permanently improve lives are what this book offers.

Some have asked me why I still have a "day job" as a Food Service Director for a school district. There are several reasons. One, I actually enjoy my school district career. Two, I enjoy being part of a team and believe I have a positive influence. Three, I rely on the income to support my family so that I don't rely on selling fitness gizmos and tall tales. When I promote healthiness part time through my speeches and books, any income gained is a bonus. I can tell the truth without holding back. I don't have to say what people *want* to hear. I get to say what they *need* to hear and my family still has a roof over their head. The benefit for you is that you can be assured that I will always tell you what I believe is best, even if it does not fatten my wallet.

That being said, how can we tell what equipment is the real deal and what will rob your healthiness zeal? Which are fitness fairy tales and which are legitimate home gyms? I will offer some guidance, but feel free to e-mail me if you are still uncertain. I personally would avoid any equipment that:

- *Only targets certain body parts*. Equipment that focuses only on your abs, thighs, butt etc. is suspect. You want equipment that can truly work your entire body. The body is a system.
- *Promises amazing results in as little as 3 minutes a day*. It is a little tough to pinpoint a time period but expect to spend at least 15 minutes a day or 30 minutes every other day to reach your goals. Anything less, consistently, and your results will be marginal.
- *Does not allow for progressive strengthening of the body*. As you will learn in later chapters, unless the body is continually challenged by progressively strengthening it, you really will never get very far. Equipment that only offers an aerobic component and promises to be a "fat burner" is not giving you the best option. True, the aerobic effect is better than sitting on your duff and is important. But significant, noticeable improvement takes place when you add the strength factor as well. Some equipment has one or two rubber bands or allows you to resist against your body weight. If that is the case, you may as well save your money and do pushups and bodyweight squats. (Not a bad idea and its free!) The good equipment I have seen on television offers between 200-400 pounds of resistance. That is enough to help most of us get somewhere.
- *Is cheap*. This is another tough one to pin down, but the old axiom; "You get what you pay for" rings loud and clear here. A great home gym can be an excellent investment. I would suggest that you avoid "cheap" if at all possible. Purchase something that is well made and will last the rest of your life.

Chapter 3

Diet Pills . . . Legalized Lying and Some are Dying

After speaking for over three hours at a conference in Florida, I returned to my hotel room and decided to turn on the television. I felt good about how the day had gone. I had presented to about 900 people, talking and teaching on fundamental health, fitness and wellness realities. The audience seemed responsive and eager to apply some of the newfound truth to their lives. It was now time for a little relaxation, and I was hoping there might be a good game or movie on the television. Perhaps you can imagine my dismay, when the very first thing to pop on the screen was an infomercial for the latest diet pill. Several things struck me as I paused to watch them spin their web. First, I wondered how anyone could believe this garbage? Secondly, I began to see how they could, as the testimonials and before and after pictures were so convincing and well done. Finally, because I know all too well who will buy these pills, I wondered how those selling these pills sleep at night.

This particular commercial was so slick. I have to admit, I was impressed with their cunningness. The commercial started out, "if you only have 5-10 pounds to lose, this product is not for you, this product is intended *only* for those who need to lose 20, 30 40 pounds or more!" That immediately qualifies over half of the countries population! It got better though. The commercial stated, "You may wonder why our product is so expensive compared to others (a one month supply is over $125.) The reason, they argue, is that their product actually works because of their secret high quality ingredients. Of course, they offer the infamous "money back guarantee". The reason these companies offer these guarantees is that they know the vast majority of people will never return a product, no matter how unhappy they are with it. I also have to believe that many people don't return these products because they don't want to admit they were gullible enough to fall for it in the first place. I have also heard through the grapevine that when people do try to return diet products, they are given the red tape run around, and made to feel like it was their fault the product did not work.

Speaking of fault, I recently heard a diet pill commercial where a so-called doctor says, "If you're overweight, it's not your fault! Rather, it is due to a harmful chemical brought on by stress that causes your body to store fat". His product, of course, takes care of all that for you. Wow. This is a form of legalized lying. The good doctor is including a *smidgen* of truth in his commercial. Yes, stress, *along* with an inactive lifestyle and poor eating habits can cause us to gain unneeded pounds. But the solution is not, never has and *never will* be in a pill or potion. Give me a break. If we needed pills to be nutritionally successful, they would grow on trees, on a bush or in the ground. A new lifestyle is what is needed. And that lifestyle is our own personal responsibility. If we are out of shape or overweight, blaming stress, or something or someone else is a copout. We have got to make a change for good and for the better. Almost every diet gimmick, fitness gizmo and weight loss company will tell you that eventually, somewhere in the tiny print, after they've convinced you that it will be much easier to make these changes with their product.

As you may notice, I am somewhat appalled at what is going on in the field of healthiness. From potions that promise you will "lose weight in your sleep while you skip exercise without skipping your favorite foods" to products and pills that say you are the "victim of a stress hormone", it is disturbing what is being sold to people as health solutions. Not only is it legalized lying, but also some are actually dying from such products. Phen-fen was finally pulled from the market and at this writing, ephedrine is finally being banned in this country after numerous deaths, strokes and other serious side effects.

I suppose that the marketers of these products are not "guilty" for selling such health solutions, as the public seems to stampede to the newest one offered. And therein lies a serious problem that you will notice mentioned throughout the book. Something has gone terribly wrong when the desire and expectation of multitudes is to get great results the quick, easy, and passive way. That desire, while understandable, will *never* work.

Most health, fitness and wellness books do not go to this length in their discussion of these negative deceptions. I do because I have seen far too many people distracted and discouraged by prevailing lies. My overriding motivation is to help you finally succeed. After more than twenty years of working with others and having had thousands of discussions on this topic, I've gained some insight into why people are failing. I believe, ultimately, it is because they have been passive in their approach. Any solution in which you are not required to move your own body on a consistent basis, while improving your eating and related health habits is passive and second rate at best. If you want to take diet pills or some other miraculous potion, the only benefit I see is that of being a placebo. Perhaps it will motivate you to work out harder and eat better because you don't want to feel like you are wasting your money. But if you have no intention of exercising and improving your nutrition, send your money to a good charity rather than wasting it on a diet pill, at least that may help improve someone's life.

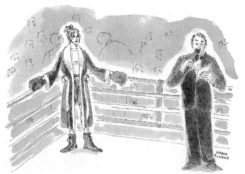

"And, in this corner, weighing five pounds more than she'd like . . . "

Chapter 4

Weight Loss Companies . . .

the Fine Art of Fine Print

Several years ago, I heard Dr. Fred Hatfield speak at a personal trainer's seminar. Dr. Hatfield is the author of several fitness and nutrition books, and a world record holder in power lifting events. He told the audience that most of the major weight loss companies in America were once sued by the federal government (FDA) for false advertising. It seems that the government's concern was that these weight loss companies were misleading customers to believe that their weight loss results would be permanent. The facts however indicated otherwise. According to Hatfield, a study was conducted of these weight loss companies. The Food and Drug Administration found that of those people that followed a commercial weight loss program and actually "lost weight", 90% gained back all that they had lost (and then some), within in a year or so.

Next time you see a weight loss company's advertisement on television, look closely for the fine print. At the bottom of the screen, in tiny fine print you will see the sentence, "**results not typical**". I think it should also say, "and most likely not permanent". Why aren't the results typical? I'll explain in more detail in a future chapter. But it boils down to this. When someone "loses weight" without maintaining or adding muscle, they will lose up to 30% of that weight in muscle which lowers their metabolism. They are now required to eat a reduced amount of calories for the rest of their life if they hope to maintain that weight. Not only is that virtually impossible for anyone to do for long, but the muscle loss is also harmful to their health. The amount of muscle on your body may be the single most important safeguard to your health, and losing any of it is NOT in your best interest.

Either the weight loss companies don't know the value of muscle or they don't want you to know. Why not? Because maintaining or building muscle requires work, and telling people they might have to work doesn't sell well in the competitive marketplace. More recently, I have seen some of the weight loss solution companies informing their clients about the importance of muscle. They are to be applauded. But the biggest names in the weight loss industry are still not doing very well in this arena. Instead, they simply tell their customers that they would benefit from "exercise" along with following their program. They do not get specific about what type of exercise is best, nor, to my knowledge, do they have assistance available to help people develop an exercise program that meets their needs. Instead, they offer vague suggestions regarding exercise, have small support group meetings, or teach their customers to count points.

I have first hand knowledge of the results such systems deliver having worked with many people who took the "weight loss company" route. Two close friends of mine lost a TON of weight in their first few months on such a program. I asked both of them if they had been taught anything at all about the importance of muscle and specific types of exercise. They replied that they had not, and in my mind, I predicted their inevitable fate. Almost one year to the date later, they had put ALL the weight back on and more!

Another couple I know is currently following a food-focused program. They diligently attend their meetings and count their points and both have lost weight. But, both complain about feeling and looking flabby. Because they are losing muscle *and* getting smaller, they now have a greater percentage of fat on their smaller bodies. No wonder they feel and look just as flabby as when they were larger. Though they have achieved becoming smaller, they are not truly healthier, fitter, stronger or more energetic. My guess is that, without actively pursuing the correct type of exercise, this couple will not be successful at keeping the weight off. And we haven't even addressed the issue of what they are eating to lose this weight!

These companies should teach you to eat and thrive with *real* food, not with points or packages. You should learn about the best types and amounts of protein, carbs, fats, vitamins, and minerals without having to depend on their companies and its products for the rest of your life. At the same time, these companies should tell and teach you that starting and saying with an effective, specific exercise program is the first and most important step towards real, permanent and effective FAT loss and a truly lean and healthy body. If you find a company or individual that does that for you, you are indeed fortunate, and I believe you will find success.

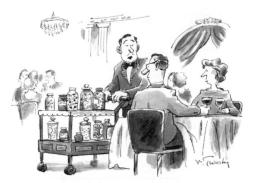

"Something from the supplement cart?"

Chapter 5

Health Food Stores . . .

Do They Have the Cure?

Occasionally I shop at the health food store. I particularly like to pick up dry roasted almonds and Odwalla fruit bars. Once in a while, I may even buy a protein bar. However, during the past few years, I've noticed subtle and disturbing changes. Frequently, I have seen hunched over, ill looking senior citizens pile up bottles of "health" solutions, herbs, and powders and then forking over $50.-$100 for these concoctions. I could be wrong, but my guess, based upon their slow gate and less than ideal posture, is that these folks are making these purchases in an effort to salvage their health. Of course, it is understandable that they want to improve their condition. But, as I witness this sight, I have to wonder if they are currently following a fitness lifestyle that includes an effective exercise and eating system, while avoiding excessive medications, stimulants, alcohol, and tobacco products. If they not following such a lifestyle, then it is quite certain that they are wasting their money.

Yes, it is better that they ingest products from the health food store as opposed to alcohol and cigarettes, but here is the issue with the health food store as cure premise. These people (and others) are hoping to purchase salvation from their poor health situation. They have likely tried traditional medicines and have been disappointed. Time and again, I have seen an elderly couple walk into the store and ask a health food store clerk about an herb or ingredient recommended as a cure. Usually, the couple asks about a product and then the clerk tells them about its wonderful qualities and the miraculous effect it can have on the body. At that point, the hopeful and encouraged couple purchase the product and head off into the wild blue yonder. But are they any better off? I really don't think so. Again, I am an optimist and like to focus on the positive. However, I have yet to hear *any* clerk ask about a person's current healthiness lifestyle habits. No, I do not spend all day hanging out at the health food store listening in on conversations. And with a few exceptions, the clerk's look reasonably healthy and fit at the store I frequent. But in regards to their knowledge and ability to actually help people who are seeking an improvement in their health, I am unconvinced.

In my utopian dreams, the conversation would go as follows: Customer asks about a product. Clerk asks why they are seeking that product, and what they hope it will accomplish. Customer states their desired goal. Clerk then asks if they are following a current, consistent exercise program that includes strength and endurance exercise. Clerk explains that such a program is the foundation to better health in that it has a profoundly positive impact on virtually every cell and system in the body. They go on to explain that by stimulating the body's cells and systems, the body becomes hungry for nutrients and good food in order to meet its energy demands and to heal, repair and grow new cells and muscle fibers. This "hunger' of the body is best met by eating real, wholesome foods with a balance of macronutrients (protein, fat, carbs) consisting of 5-8 smaller, equally sized meals every three hours or so. The clerk then informs the customer that if they are smoking cigarettes or drinking in excess, they are really screwing up their system. Any products they buy will not do any good when such toxins are circulating in their body. At that point, it would be fine to sell the customer what they want to purchase. But to sell them high-priced hope in a bottle as a way to treat their condition without informing them that quality foods and exercise are necessary for the product to be of any value, is misleading and a disservice.

The same is true of other types of customers I have seen in health food stores. Don't get me wrong. I shop at the health food store, along with other fit, reasonably well-adjusted, healthy people. But it is safe to say the following. The majority of those visiting health food stores these days are either seeking the latest cure, looking to lose weight or hoping to build muscle. I will spare you the entire song and dance again, but the point is the same. Whether a customer is seeking the latest diet pill or a skinny teenage guy is looking for the latest, greatest supplement to get buffed, both are wasting their time and money unless they have a foundational fitness and health lifestyle in place. You may ask, is it really the responsibility of the health food store to educate their customers? That depends upon whether they really want to help others or just make a buck. So shop and buy, as you desire at the health food store. Just realize that supplements *alone* aren't the cure or the ticket to ultimately reaching the healthiness shore.

Chapter 6

Thigh Cream and Other Dreams

As we prepare to wrap up this section of the book, let's pay a brief visit to some of the most absurd and ridiculous "items of the day". No, I am not promoting Bill O'Reilly. But this phrase he coined is perfect for describing these last few "gems" of fraud. It appears almost unfathomable that these items would actually get to the marketplace and sell, but oh well. Maybe I should still consider the production of "Freddie the Fitness Frog". I mean if people will buy thigh cream, why not?

Thigh cream has been on the market for several years now. At first it was marketed with outrageous claims like "watch your thighs disappear in front of your eyes". Now, well-known companies are marketing it with more subdued claims of, "Up to 1" thinner thighs in 4 weeks flat! Introducing . . . the worst thing to happen to cellulite since the treadmill!" Another add on the Internet is more aggressive. Its advertisement reads, "Get The Smooth, Sleek and Sexy Beauty of Cover Girl Thighs Like These IN JUST 3 SHORT WEEKS—Without Doing A Single Leg Raise . . . Cycling A Single Mile . . . Or Jogging A Single Step! AND NO DIETING

EITHER! Simply cream on this new doctor-developed, MIRACLE THIGH CREAM, called "Product X"—and in JUST 21 DAYS, *or even less*, see the entire area from your hips to your knees magically transformed into the most flattering feature of your entire figure." Sounds good doesn't it? Recently, however, I read this report from the National Council Against Health Fraud:

THIGH CREAM FAILS TESTS: Washington University researchers found that the highly publicized aminophylline-containing thigh cream does not work. Dr. Leroy Young, professor of plastic and reconstructive surgery, studied 17 women who massaged either the cream or a placebo into one thigh and one side of their stomach for a period of four weeks. Eleven women completed the study (the others dropped out when they saw no improvement). Curiously, one woman was convinced that the cream worked for her even though her weight and measurements were unchanged! "Some people just believe in miracles," said Young.

Miracles *are* possible. By following the steps in this book, you may well experience what some would consider a miracle makeover of your health, fitness and appearance. It will require intelligent effort, discipline, and some time. I assure you, the results will be well worth it, they will be real results you can take pride and have confidence in.

Another absurd and ridiculous item of the day is the recently banished "electronic abs stimulator". Perhaps you saw this on television before it was yanked for false advertising. You simply attached some pads to your stomach and turned it on to let it exercise your abs. You just relaxed while your belly just vaporized. The good news is that this product and its promoter are facing charges for fraudulent advertising. The bad news, once again, is that their advertisements were extremely convincing and they sold thousands of them!

Another very suspect practice is "cleansing". Over the past few years, I have had several people bring up the topic of cleansing. At a recent conference, a woman asked me if she should get a cleansing before starting a fitness program. A man last week (whose wife heard me speak over a year ago) told me he thinks she needs a cleansing before she does anything. Personally, I think that if a person starts living the lifestyle in this book, they will get all the cleansing they need. It will come in the form of good old-fashioned sweat. And, in my informed opinion, that is all the cleansing anyone needs. I think much of the cleansing focus is from people who want to avoid the real thing and any real work. If everybody in America would focus on intentionally breaking a little sweat each day through an effective exercise program, our whole health and fitness problem would start getting "cleaned" up right away. For too many, cleansings represent another way of deluding themselves into thinking that there must be a secret or an easier way.

I am sure this chapter will grow in length over the years. As long as people continue to look for the magic dust of healthiness magic, we can be sure someone will be happily waving their magic wand and saying to us, "abra kadabra . . . hocus pocus . . . give me your $$$$$$". None too soon, the federal government is getting more aggressive in reining in the snake oil peddlers of dangerous diet drugs, misleading advertisements, and supplements that claim to be a cure all. And thankfully, we can always count on traditional health care to help us break free and enjoy greater health. Or can we?

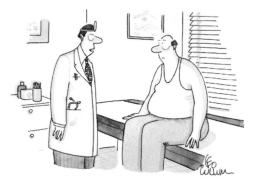

"Your skin is enlarged."

Chapter 7

Health Care or Sick Care?

Doctor, Doctor, Give Me the News . . .

Sal Arria, co-founder of the International Sport Sciences Association (where I received my first fitness certification) and a Chiropractor, asks the question, "Why is our medical system called health care?" His argument is that it should rightfully be called "sick care", as that is its primary function. Hospitals, doctors, etc, are involved in the treatment of people who are experiencing sickness, not health. Hospitals are filled with sick and injured people, not healthy ones. Make no mistake. This is a needed service. People do get sick, have accidents, etc. and need help to get better. My aim is not to be negative or disrespectful to doctors. Like you, my family and I have personally benefited from the care of highly skilled, professional, trustworthy and caring doctors. If I were in a car accident on the way home today, I would want a capable doctor and a good hospital available to take care of me. I am quite sure that my loved ones will need and benefit from the services of a doctor, hospital, or health clinic in the future. But I am equally certain that most doctors agree that critical aspects of our traditional "health" care system are flawed.

Dr. Arria's primary concern with doctors and the "sick" care system is that doctors are quick to prescribe medications and surgeries, but rarely do they prescribe fitness. In the case of patients with poor health and chronic diseases, fitness is ultimately what they need. Most surgeries, medications and prescriptions will never be able to improve a person's health like a fitness lifestyle can. This situation, while not good, can be explained. Doctors are *trained* to do three primary things: diagnose, prescribe or perform surgery. Those are their overall functions, role and responsibility. And, in some cases, that is what a person needs. But when this is not the case, they remain limited to those options.

How can I make such comments as a mere fitness trainer? Well, let me just give you one example. I recently had the pleasure of helping a gentleman improve his fitness levels. When I met him, he was on three different medications, primarily to help with digestive issues and high blood pressure. His doctor had prescribed these medications for him. In my opinion, what the doctor should have prescribed was a fitness lifestyle implemented with the help of a certified personal trainer. Why? Because the gentleman in question was carrying approximately 60 lbs. of excess body fat and *not* involved in an effective exercise program at the time. Medications all have a direct and often negative impact on a person, and they do NOTHING to help with the foundational issues of living in an unfit body. Why don't most doctors prescribe fitness programs? Perhaps malpractice lawsuits are to blame. But many physicians don't realize the value of fitness, perhaps don't know where to refer a patient to, or feel hindered, as insurance may not cover the cost. One also has to wonder if some don't prescribe fitness, simply because it is not profitable to them.

These statements are not true of all doctors, clinics, and hospitals. Around the country, more and more hospitals are building health clubs/gyms adjacent to their hospital, as they understand that patients will not really get better until they take up a new lifestyle. In my hometown, there are a few doctors who are prescribing fitness and insurance companies are now beginning to pay for these services. These are good and necessary developments.

The gentleman spoken of earlier ended up losing approximately 35 pounds of that excess fat, dropping all three medications, and lowering his blood pressure. This took less than six months, simply by applying *some* of the concepts in this book. The truth is that his results were marginal compared to what he could achieve if he fully committed himself. This is especially true when it comes to following the nutritional recommendations. Even with less than total commitment, he made better health and fitness progress than any pill, medication or surgery could have provided. With better adherence, his results would have been even more remarkable. I am sure his doctor is a man of integrity and a consummate, caring professional. My question, though, is why did he not help this gentleman adopt a fitness lifestyle sooner?

The doctors do not completely share the blame for this situation. They have to make a living and sending people to gyms and trainers may not pay the bills. In some ways, their hands are tied as pharmaceutical drug companies drive the "health care" system and performing surgeries is very lucrative. Been to a doctor's office lately? Every time I visit a doctor it seems like there is a pharmaceutical drug salesperson there as well, dropping off samples and tickets to the latest sports game. I have a buddy from high school who has a great career. He visits doctor's offices, wines and dines them at major sporting events and then wins all expense paid trips to exotic getaways for his sales efforts. Is he to blame? No, I don't think it's that simple. There is BIG money in prescription drugs. Just watch the evening news one night. Last week, during one hour of the evening news I counted 8 different prescription drug commercials. These companies would argue that they are helping others and providing a valuable and needed service. I would argue that this is not true much of the time. My estimate is that at least 50% of medication prescribed and taken is unnecessary. The healthiest, safest, and most effective prescription is to improve one's lifestyle. The problem with prescription drugs is that they all have side effects and, some would even argue, a *direct* negative effect on a person's health.

While working as the coordinator of the Shasta County Health Promotion Project, I would visit the homes of senior citizens with poor health. Several of the people visited were taking as many as 8 different medications. Taking multiple medications is known as polypharmacy, and is estimated to cause as many as 100,000 deaths a year. What were these people's doctors thinking? How can that be good for anyone? Nevertheless, let's make one thing clear. *If you are on a prescription drug or are considering starting one, follow your doctor's advice.* I am not a doctor and am not saying that **all** medications at all times are bad for you. At the same time, however, show them this book. Get their approval to start making lifestyle changes with fitness and food. Then, both you and your doctor will be stepping out of the sick care cycle and into a more hopeful and helpful healthiness lifestyle. And that is what any good doctor would want!

Chapter 8

Passive versus Active . . .

Who You Gonna Call?

Several years ago, I met a family physician at the gym. He was there regularly, lifting weights and running on the treadmill. I remember discussing with him the concept of prescribing fitness to his patients, including strength training. He obviously believed in the health benefits of strength training for himself. His comment was discouraging. He said, "I tell my patients that they need to take better care of themselves, but I can't even get them to walk, let alone take up strength training". A chiropractor friend of mine echoed the same sentiment. He said that he tries to get patients to do curative exercises to strengthen their backs and bodies, but very few comply. Instead, they prefer to come in and get their backs adjusted periodically and return to their inactive lifestyles. What is he to do? He adjusts them to give them temporary relief, and then expects he will see them again in a few weeks. So, we must bear some of the blame for our less than ideal "health" care system because of our own unwillingness to comply with what responsible health care professionals recommend. The same doctor who has trouble getting his patients to walk said that most patients simply want a pill to make them feel better. In fact, some of his patients demand that he, "just give them something!"

The fact that you have read this far suggests that you want something better. It is important that you understand the concept of passive versus active treatment. Passive treatment can help you up to a point, and has its place in our lives and health. Passive treatment is, *anytime anyone else does something to or for you, and does not involve any ongoing voluntary effort on your part.* Examples of passive treatments include the services of a physician, chiropractor, physical therapist, massage therapist, acupuncturist, dietitian, and so forth. Active treatment, on the other hand, is when *we* take control of managing our own movements and motions on an ongoing and independent basis. Active treatment is when things REALLY improve, and for good. You may need assistance from a fitness professional for a time, but they don't exercise for you and ultimately, you will be the one moving yourself.

While we are still discussing this concept of passive versus active, we should address some activities that stand out as the epitome of passive. In the previous chapter, I mentioned that surgeries are lucrative. It appears that they aren't always necessary either. In my hometown a physician was found to have performed several hundred unneeded heart surgeries. The story made "Sixty Minutes" and stories like it happen all over the country. I know two guys who went to the doctor because of shoulder pain. Both received cortisone shots for pain in their shoulders and were told that surgery may be needed. In neither case did the doctor discuss therapeutic exercises that these men could try. I'm not sure why. Perhaps they didn't know what exercises would help or maybe they were concerned about malpractice suits, which I suppose is understandable. The bummer though, is these men did not receive assistance that would help them in the long-run. The only option for a "cure" was to go under the knife. Even physical therapy would have been better than a shot but, of course, the insurance company will only cover a limited number of visits. What these men needed was direct instruction on how to treat the problem area themselves without surgery and, hopefully, without shots. For instance, several years ago, my father-in-law complained to me of severe shoulder pain. He was driving a truck cross-country at the time. I showed him a simple external rotation exercise he could do in the truck with a small amount of weight. According to him, after several weeks, the pain was gone. He's retired from driving now. But, should the pain return, he knows how to take care of it himself.

Whether or not various types of surgeries are performed needlessly in great numbers, I am not sure. However, there are two types of surgeries that I think are unnecessary. The first is gastrointestinal bypass, otherwise known as "stomach stapling". I have been surprised to learn of the increasing number of people having this procedure. Some of these people are near and dear to me and I understand, that for some of them, their bodyweight has been a difficult struggle for many, many years. I also happen to know that these same individuals have not exercised or eaten right for significant periods of time. I'm sure that doctors make very good money on these surgeries, and insurance companies may be covering them. But these surgeries do not address the real issue. If a person cannot control their eating or consistently exercise, they have a deeper problem that needs to be addressed. To me, getting your stomach stapled (or wrapped) is like driving down the road and noticing the oil light comes on. You pull over to the side of the road, lift the hood, find the wire going to the oil light, and cut the wire so that the oil light goes off.

The root of the problem is not corrected. It is also expensive, has a degree of risk, and is not guaranteed to work. It does, however, make certain doctors wealthy and they will be pleased to do it for you. In fact, a recent television special outlined the dangers of stomach stapling and reviewed several cases where the results were not only negative, but nearly life threatening. In virtually every case, the patient was **told** that they *needed* the surgery because their current condition of obesity was life threatening. No kidding. It took a doctor to figure that out? Personally, I think that sounds like a scam that paid for the physician's beachfront home. If someone you know is even considering this as an option, I suggest you encourage them to implement the lifestyle recommended in this book for one year first. Yes, stomach stapling is much faster and "easier" but it is not without significant and long-term health risks. And without exercise, those electing this option will simply become a smaller, flabby person. In regards to fitness and health, faster and easier is NOT best. So many adults complain about the young people of today being lazy and unmotivated. But haven't we set a precedent for fast, short cut, whiny, no effort living? Our lifestyle choices not only affect our physical body, but also the fiber of our character.

There is a way that you can achieve healthier results and increase your self-image at the same time. Take up and live the lifestyle taught in this book. If you have already had the surgery, please implement these healthiness concepts right away. That way you can be assured that it is because of *your* active efforts, self-discipline and self-control that your body and mindset will *stay* healthy, fit and strong for the remainder of your life.

Another surgery that is growing in popularity is thyroid surgery. I have talked with dozens of people over the past few years that are considering thyroid surgery. In nearly every case the person was a woman in their 30's or 40's who felt that their low energy levels and continual weight gain was due to a thyroid problem. In *every* single instance, not *one* of these people was living a healthiness lifestyle. These were people I knew personally and I was aware of their eating habits. Each confessed that they were not following *any* exercise program. I am convinced that their lifestyle was contributing to a slow metabolism, depression, low energy and weight gain, not their thyroid! Yet their doctors were ready to yank that sucker out, without having thoroughly examined the weaknesses of their current health practices.

We *create* our unique metabolism by our lifestyle and by how much muscle we carry on our body. Hopefully your doctor will tell you the same rather than perform a surgery you may not need. Diligently follow a program like the one in this book before even considering thyroid or stomach surgery. Follow the path of active vs. passive treatment and you will be on your way to astonishing healthiness.

Section III

Looking for Lean in All the Wrong Places!!

No one needs to be hopeless when it comes to healthiness, because it's what we're made of that matters.

Chapter 9

Fishing in the Sahara

Depression is at epidemic proportions in this country. According to the World Health Organization, by the year 2025, depression will be the most diagnosed health issue in this country. Well, that is depressing news, and really unnecessary. Depression, you see, is something I know a little about. I once spent three and a half years in a psychiatric hospital. I was working there as the director of Nutrition Services. We used to have training sessions on the various issues affecting our patients so that we could better serve them. We frequently studied depression. What stood out to me was that depression is often rooted in hopelessness. Fortunately, when it comes to our healthiness, we do not need to be hopeless or depressed, despite the obstacles and roadblocks. We actually have the key to better healthiness inside our own human body and it begins with understanding the miracle of muscle.

If "miracle" sounds too dramatic for you, consider Webster's definition: "an event or action that contradicts known scientific laws." What do we accept as scientific law in this country? What is conventional thinking in regards to our health, fitness, and wellness? Conventional thinking is that as we get a little older, we must get a little weaker, a little slower, a little fatter, a little sicker, and then 10, 20, 30, 40 and even 50 years ahead of schedule we become "victims" of poor health and live out the rest of our lives in that state. This thinking does not just apply to older people. The majority of younger Americans also qualify as being in abysmal shape. Statistics are showing that younger and younger people are being diagnosed with chronic diseases such as diabetes due to their inactive lifestyles and poor food choices.

It does not have to be this way. As you will soon learn, you can get a miracle makeover in your life by simply adding more muscle to your body. This is a fact that should be shouted from the rooftops by medical, health and fitness professions everywhere. Consider this next statement thoughtfully and carefully. **Nearly every single, serious, physical health issue that we face in this country boils down to the lack of muscle on a person's body, in combination with excess body fat.**

Trying to improve your health, bodyweight or wellness without focusing on muscle is like trying to catch fish without a fishing pole in the Sahara! Your chances of success aren't great. But the predominant emphasis in this country for over twenty years has been on fat, fat, fat. We hear very little about the need for more muscle on our bodies. But it is the lack of muscle that drives unhealthy hearts, poor digestive and nervous systems, weak bones, bad backs, poor posture, weak knees, lowered immunity, poor eating habits and the accumulation of fat. Having too little muscle is the ultimate health problem for the vast majority of Americans. If everyone had more of what fitness expert Phil Kaplan calls a "concern for muscle", the number of people impacted by lifestyle diseases (i.e., high blood pressure, diabetes) could be dramatically reduced.

Maintaining, building and restoring muscle (lean tissue) on our bodies *demands* that we pay close attention to how we live. That is why I continually harp about the healthiness lifestyle concept. At the very core of the "healthiness habit" is a focus on maintaining the proper amount of muscle on your body. If you do this, keeping off excess body fat will naturally occur and virtually all of your bodies systems and related organs will function at an optimum level and for the longest time possible.

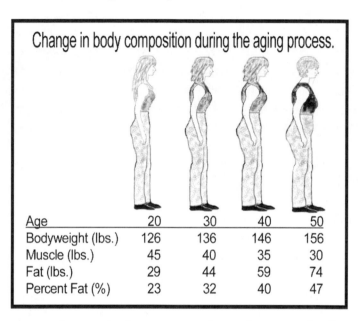

Change in body composition during the aging process.

Age	20	30	40	50
Bodyweight (lbs.)	126	136	146	156
Muscle (lbs.)	45	40	35	30
Fat (lbs.)	29	44	59	74
Percent Fat (%)	23	32	40	47

Because we ignore the importance of muscle on our bodies, we allow this incredibly valuable health resource to dissipate over the decades and then wonder why our health is declining. In a few moments, I will delineate the details of what makes muscle such a miracle maker in maintaining marvelous health. First, we need to take a look at what happens to the typical person in this country. This particular image uses a woman, but the same phenomenon occurs with men. With men however, the weight usually appears in different places.

Notice that the woman on the left, at 20 years of age, had a bodyweight of 126 pounds and carried 45 pounds of muscle on her body. Look at what happens each decade as she ages. Every 10 years, she has let about 5 pounds of life preserving muscle leave her body. By age fifty, she carries only 30 pounds of muscle. Her fat weight went from 29 pounds at age 20 to a whopping 74 pounds at age fifty and the percentage of fat on her body increased from 23% to 47%. These figures are the results of studies done with average people. These findings represent our nations single greatest contributor to poor health. This is what prevents so many from enjoying the benefits of feeling and looking great throughout the majority of their life. The GOOD news is that the above scenario is completely reversible! We can actually return to what we had in your youth simply by adopting a lifestyle that restores muscle. The woman above could physically return to what she had at 20. And you can do the same.

"But Muscle!! I don't want muscle! I don't want to get all big and buffed!" These are the comments I hear ALL the time, mostly from women, but occasionally from men. These types of comments beg the question, "If you don't want muscle, what do you want?" The typical response I hear is that they would like to get "**toned and fit.**" O.K. Clearly, it is time for a quick anatomy lesson.

The human body is made up of essentially five components. They include water, organs, fat, bones and muscle. If you don't want more muscle, what do you want more of? Do you want more water? Not unless you are dehydrated. Do you want more organs? Probably not unless you are missing one! Do you want more fat? Most of us don't need anymore. Do you want more bone? Maybe, most of us could stand to add a little more bone. But, the BEST way to get more bone is through weight bearing exercise that first builds more muscle.

The big scare for women in regards to muscle is that it might give them muscles like a man, making them appear less feminine. I thought this age old myth had long since been removed, but still hear it everywhere I go. If this is a concern of yours, please understand, the overwhelming majority of women *cannot* build muscles like a man. Women do not naturally posses the amount of testosterone needed to have the size and strength of male muscles.

Successful women bodybuilders are a combination of rare genetics, intensive, often lengthy and specially designed workouts, extremely low body fat, and yes, sometimes the use of hormone enhancing chemical substances (steroids). The same is true with men bodybuilders. Very few of us could ever look like these people, **even if we wanted to** and no matter how hard we worked. The great majority of us simply do not have the God given genetics. Thinking that you could start lifting weights and end up looking like a bodybuilder is like thinking that, if you play a lot of basketball, you could end up 7 feet tall!

If size is your concern, you may not understand what I call the *Miracle Making Properties of Muscle.* Miracle making property #1 is that a pound of muscle on the human body is about 1/5 the size of a pound of fat. Said another way, a pound of fat on the human body is approximately 5 times larger than a pound of muscle. Muscle does not make you bigger; it actually will make you smaller. It makes you more compact. As far as appearance goes, Marilyn Monroe's beauty secret was weight lifting. She understood that maintaining muscle is what enhances a women's feminine figure. Thousands, if not millions, of women are now learning and benefiting from this principle. My wife showed me an episode of Oprah that focused on the benefits of strength training for women. The show featured a mother of nine who was in top condition, attractive and feminine. She stated that strength training is the key to staying young. It is her fountain of youth that allows her to handle the demands of her family. She said that if a woman wants the best for her health and appearance, stimulating muscle growth is the goal. Likewise, if a man is concerned about his appearance, muscle certainly looks better than fat. Interestingly, the children of this mom were interviewed and asked how they felt about their "weight lifting" mom. The kids were proud of her and remarked how nice it was to have a mom who could actually play and keep up with them! They were proud of how good she looked, especially for a forty-something mom with nine children.

Jan Todd, co-author of the book, *Lift Your Way to Youthful Fitness* says, "Women should not be so concerned about what will happen to them if they *do* lift weights, rather, they should be concerned about what will happen to them if they *don't.*"

The primary focus of this book is not about appearance. The focus is healthiness. Appearances improve as a result of that focus. The miracle making property of muscle really moves the mountains that can prevent healthiness. Fitness and strength author Wayne Westcott, P.H.D. calls muscle the "engine" of the body. Phil Kaplan, whom I quoted earlier, calls muscles the, "batteries of the body". The more muscle a person carries, relative to body fat and body weight, the more power, stamina, and health they will have.

Miracle making property #2 is that muscle is *ALIVE!!* Muscle is the primary component of what is known as, "metabolically active mass". Just one pound of muscle on the human body burns 50-90 calories per day. A pound of fat burns only 2 calories per day. Muscle fiber is packed with mitochondria, which produces ATP, which are like little furnaces in our body that create and consume energy. Adding muscle is like adding firepower to your body. It makes doing everything easier and reduces the strain on your heart, lungs, bones, joints, tendons, and more. Excess fat is virtually dead weight. It drags you down, makes you tired, wears you out and places additional, sometimes deadly strain on your entire body.

Earlier we discussed diet pills. One of the big claims of diet pills is that they will speed up your metabolism, and have a "thermogenic" effect. Depending on the ingredients, that could be true. The problem is that this effect is temporary, could damage your heart, may create an addiction and will leave you drained and probably depressed when it wears off. The best way to permanently and safely increase your metabolism is to add muscle to your body. By doing so, it creates what author Nick Nillson calls a permanent, "metabolic surge". The amount of muscle on our bodies is BY FAR the #1 determinant of our metabolism. According to the Keiser Institute of Aging, an increase of only 7.7% in the resting metabolic rate of a 180-pound person can result in an increase of 50,000 calories expended yearly. This can result in a loss of 14 pounds of fat even if diet and daily activity remain constant.

Here's how that could work for you. Imagine that you had an identical twin. Just for illustration, lets say you both have the physical measurements of the 50-year-old woman in the chart above. You both weigh 156 pounds, have 30 pounds of muscle and carry 74 pounds of fat on your body. Then, someone who cares a lot about you gives you this book. Being the wise person that you are, you decide to adopt the suggested techniques of the book into your lifestyle. Fast-forward with me one year. Your twin, who did nothing different for the past year, still weighs 156, has 30 pounds of muscle and 74 pounds of fat. You, on the other hand, have *added* 10 pounds of muscle **while** *losing* 10 pounds of fat. Remember, you still both weigh 156 pounds. But here's the cool news. Because you have added 10 pounds of muscle, you now burn an additional 500-900 calories per day, every day, 356 days per year, seven days a week, even when you sleep (remember, each pound of muscle burns 50-90 calories per day). You can eat between 500-900 calories more per day without gaining fat and everything on your body is working more effectively. Your clothes fit better because you have lost inches (1lb. of fat is 5x larger than 1lb. of muscle), you look and feel better and have more energy to do the things you want to do. Your immune system, balance, confidence, and ability to handle stress have been also been enhanced.

Don't Go Outside Naked!

Life is better and brighter when you have more muscle. Muscle has been called the engine, batteries and life preserver of the body. With that in mind, it might be the most important physical "clothing" you will ever wear. It is what separates the sick from the healthy, the physically frail from the strong and vibrant, the lean from the obese, and the weary from the high geared. Think about someone you know who is in bad health. It is their appearance that first catches our attention. We become concerned about a loved one who begins losing weight and getting weak because we know this is a sign that they are losing strength and the fight for life. Or the opposite may be true. We smell trouble when someone's body weight seems out of control. Muscle is buried and then lost while their body grows larger and stresses under the load.

Perhaps your concern is more similar to our fifty-year-old friend who is facing progressive muscle loss, fat gain and diminishing health. We can stop this unfriendly process in its tracks and progressively reverse it by focusing on restoring muscle and reducing excess body fat. You will learn the most effective ways to do this in the next section of the book. But I will tell you now; it is going to be something you will need to focus on each day if you are going to enjoy its benefits. It's kind of like getting dressed every day.

Have you ever thought about how much time you spend every morning getting dressed? For some, it may only be a few minutes, for others perhaps 45 minutes to over an hour. But one thing we know, in our society, everyone gets dressed before they go outside to work, shopping etc. No matter how stressed or late we are, we always make time to put our clothes on. This is a good thing. I had a neighbor once who decided to mow his lawn with no clothes on. I never saw him again after that day. True story. The point is that we always make time to get dressed, because we believe and accept that we must. It is a priority that we do not challenge.

If you *REALLY* want exclusively good health, now and throughout your life, you are going to have to view exercise in the same light. It is so crucial to extraordinary health and living that it cannot be negotiated. Allow me to illustrate in another way. What would happen if we didn't brush and floss our teeth daily? At first, it would just feel a little gross. Can you imagine not brushing and flossing your teeth for several days at a time? You know what would happen. Things would get pretty nasty quickly. The same thing is happening inside of us when we fail to exercise our bodies properly each day. Gunk starts building up on the insides, and eventually works it's way through the body and shows up on the outside of the body.

From this day forward, it is my hope that as you dress yourself each day, this concept will stick in your brain. May you be reminded that you should reserve time each day to "brush and floss" the insides of your wonderfully and awesomely made body through effective physical exercise. Your insides and your outside will work and feel better. I know it is tough to find the time. As this book goes on, I will challenge you to evaluate how you spend time. I will share some ideas on how you can get more time out of your day. It really doesn't take *that* much time. Remember, when it comes to your health and exercise, "don't go outside naked". Dress yourself with the clothing that will never go out of fitness fashion: a healthy, life-giving coat of muscle. To wear this coat through the seasons of your life and reap a harvest of healthiness means that you will need to continuously take time to plant the seeds of effective exercise.

Chapter 10

Losing Weight Can Make You a Smaller, Fatter, and Sicker Person!

"Did you hear about Billy Bob and Sally Jane? They lost umpteen pounds on the "you-fill-in-the-blank" diet, they *look* so good." While many see the fact that someone has been able to lose weight as good news, such is not always the case. Looks can be quite deceiving. For many in diet-only-mania-land, the "look" they achieve is usually just a temporary and illusionary picture of health and fitness.

Remember the chart of the women who lost muscle and gained fat as she aged? Most people try to correct that dilemma by going on a diet to "lose weight". But make no mistake; *diets alone* are doomed to fail! In the food and nutrition section of this book, more detail is given on how you can make healthy food choices, but before we can utilize that information, we must first overcome destructive behaviors that cause despair and desperation.

Desiring to "lose weight" in order to improve health and appearance is not a step in the wrong direction. Figuring out how to best accomplish that can be a challenge. A friend recently called and said that his doctor told him he needed to lose about thirty pounds. My friend was a little miffed and seemed to want me to say that it wasn't a good idea. Given that my friend is inactive, two inches shorter than I am, has similar bone structure, is 12 years older, and outweighs me by about thirty pounds, I had to say that his doctors' prognosis seemed right on. I mentioned that rather than being upset, he should be happy to have a doctor who cares enough to tell him the truth at the risk of upsetting his patient. My friend agreed, but also noted that his doctor did not tell him **how** to lose the excess weight. Where does one begin and whom do you listen to?

In a later chapter, we will review the myriad of "diets" that are proliferating like rabbits, but for now, I want to stress that the DIET ONLY approach to weight loss leads to a large likelihood of lasting failure. You may remember that when a person loses weight, up to 25% of the pounds (or more) represent muscle loss. Because muscle is the primary driver of our metabolism, losing muscle is not a good thing. When you lower your metabolism through dieting, you must consume a restricted amount of calories to maintain your new weight. This is the reason that dieting alone is doomed to fail. No one can maintain eating a restricted amount of calories forever. Our bodies require food and we like to eat it as well.

The illustration below show what happens to a man who goes on a calorie or nutrient restricted diet alone (like Atkins). He will loose weight comprised of fat, water, muscle and bone. What he may not know is that up to 30% of his weight loss can come from muscle. The results show that he lost 50lbs., which he might think is a good thing. However, his percentage of body fat has actually increased from 25% to 30%! He is now a *smaller, fatter person*! Because he lost muscle (which burns more calories than fat), his metabolism is slower. He will have to permanently lower his caloric intake to keep from gaining weight. Eventually, he'll get tired of depriving himself and begin to increase the amount of food he eats. Slowly, all the weight will return to a body that has less muscle! When this happens, he will become a *bigger, fatter* person!

Figure A

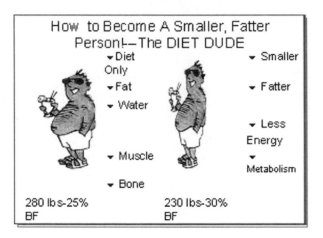

Thank goodness there is a better way. By following a lifestyle that includes eating and exercising in a healthy way, you can shed excess fat while **adding muscle** and a little bone. You will look leaner, feel stronger and be able to INCREASE food intake. As you continue with this lifestyle, your health and energy levels will constantly improve. Our friend in the picture decided to do this and had the following results.

This time the outcome is more favorable. He lost fat weight, added muscle, increased his metabolism and energy while improving his health and appearance.

Figure B

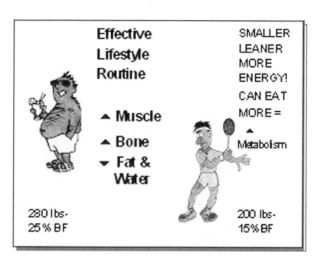

As you can see, it is crucial to maintain and build muscle through an effective exercise program while you attempt to shed excess body fat. PLEASE do not try to just "lose weight" by dieting. Set a goal to become a LFIAAWM (pronounced "lif-uh-wum"): a lean, fat-incinerating, anti-aging wellness machine! Losing weight *alone* is ultimately a foolish endeavor. Focus on losing **fat** while adding **muscle** and a little bone. One of the keys to doing this successfully will be to say good-bye to an old nemesis, or at least send it on a long vacation!

Kiss your scale goodbye!

Your scale is not your friend. Scales do not distinguish between muscle, fat, and water weight. When you initially starts the "Fit Food Lifestyle Formula" ™, you may initially *gain* "pounds" as you add muscle. This is a good thing! Remember, you are adding *batteries* to your body first so you can burn off fat. People are programmed to weigh themselves and evaluate their progress based on what the scale reads. It is sad that people are in such bondage to the scale. I always tell clients to give their scale to a friend for at least three months and forget about weighing themselves for a season. If you just won't do that and are going to weigh yourself, make sure you do it in a manner that will be encouraging rather than negative. Instead, we want to measure what really matters: body composition, otherwise known as "body fat percentage".

There are a number of ways to measure body fat percentage. The most popular way is through skin fold calipers. If you have a personal trainer, you can ask them do this for you or you can learn to do it yourself. Calipers can be purchased on my website at a small discount or you can buy them from most fitness retailers. Body fat percentage, according to the former Surgeon General, Dr. David Thatcher, is the single most important measurement of a person's health. I agree completely. Unfortunately, I have heard no other government officials emphasize body composition or body fat percentage. Most people instead focus on body mass index (height/weight ratio).

This is understandable I suppose, in that it is a much easier way to evaluate obesity. By simply looking at a person's weight and height, they can quickly estimate whether a person is obese. The BIG problem with this system is that it does not measure what a person is *made* of. A heavily muscled, thick boned individual could be evaluated as obese by using the body mass index scale. Consider Emit Smith, the future NFL Hall of fame running back. He would be classified as obese on the body mass index scale but his body fat percentage is actually very low. On the other hand, an anorexic person might appear to be within normal ranges. Yet many anorexics are actually clinically obese because they lack muscle and bone! Their starving body has consumed their muscle and they are literally all fat and bones. Just because a person *appears* thin and fit does not mean they are the models of health.

Although the expense and impracticality of taking body fat measurements could be cumbersome, the government, mass media and medical community should begin to implement this type of evaluation. This is important for several reasons. It has long been known that there are various body shapes called "soma types". Ectomorphs are naturally thin people, mesomorphs are naturally well muscled and what we consider to be well proportioned, and there are the endomorphs, who are usually thick boned and more heavyset. To ignore these differences when evaluating weight seems ridiculous. This is especially true for a person who is an endomorph (large, thick boned person). They might be quite healthy, with low body fat percentage, and ample muscle strength, but the body mass index will say that they are overweight. Discouraged, they struggle to reach standards that are unreasonable given their natural shape. I think this is especially harmful with endomorphic children, who certainly do not need to be told that they are "fat".

Body fat percentage is something that any of us can improve upon, independent of our body type, bone structure or overall size. It is what really matters. By restoring or increasing our miracle making muscle and reducing excess body fat, we can be on our way to a brighter, fitter future. So hold on to your hat, because next we will look at exactly what kind of exercise will help us do just that!

SECTION IV

Help Your Body Win!

Chapter 11

Mirror, Mirror on the Wall . . .

What Will Make Me Fittest of All??

"They are most fatigued who know not what to do"
Anonymous

We have been told for decades, that the key to maintaining our health is to "eat right and exercise". People seem to accept this and it is not uncommon to hear remarks like "walking is the best exercise" and that you should pick an exercise "that you enjoy, and that is fun". Simply focus on, "calories in versus calories out", is the advice armchair experts eagerly offer. Well, most of these comments carry a degree of truth and correctness, but they are far too general to be of much benefit to anyone.

When we are looking at this whole subject of exercise, we need to ask ourselves, what is our goal? For most considering an exercise program, the goal is to help them enjoy great health, feel really good, reduce the effects of stress, have lots of energy, live longer, be independent, be productive and capable of most physical tasks and look their absolute best. I believe that should about cover it. Let me know if I missed anything. These are great goals, but you should know that some activities are significantly better than others when it comes to improving your physical condition. Ninety out of 100 Americans *do not* have an exercise/fitness program in their lives that will help them reach the goals described. There is so much confusion about what exercises are actually helpful.

Personal fitness trainers are paid, evaluated and judged almost solely on their ability to help you sort through the confusion and get results. It helps if they are nice and you enjoy your time with them, but bottom line, you want to see improvements that are real and measurable. We can discuss exercise methods all day long, but in the end, you are going to want to know that I KNOW the absolute best methods on the planet for getting results for you. My plan to meet this need is to teach you a core group of foundational exercises that will provide the fastest, safest, and most effective results possible. If you learn these exercises and do them regularly, you will meet your goals and be independent of me (and costly trainers/programs) for the rest of your life. Sound like a good deal? Good.

Before we move on, it would be a good idea to look at a couple definitions of exercise. Webster's definition is "bodily or mental exertion, especially for the sake of training or improvement of health." Not too bad, but a little indirect for our purposes. I prefer this one from Brian D. Johnston, author of *Exercise Science: Theory & Practice*: "Vigorous muscular exertion performed with the intent of making an *inroad* (a reduction) into the body's functional ability in order to stimulate a physiological adaptive response to decelerate (slow down) the loss of, to maintain, or to improve said functional ability. I grant you that is a mouth full but the good news is that what is "vigorous" for each of us is different! Although a little technical, Mr. Johnston's definition is excellent. It is very accurate and points out what so many exercise experts seem to be missing when making recommendations of methods.

The bottom line is this: "If you want *to make a noticeable difference*, choose exercises that temporarily *mess* up your physiology in a significant but safe way." When you lift weights, you break down your muscle fibers. You take a day off between workouts to allow your body to rest. During that time, your muscle fibers will **recreate** and repair themselves making them stronger and healthier. Each time you workout and follow-up with a rest period, this process occurs. As a result, your muscular system (and entire body including the nervous system, heart, vascular system, etc.) is forced to continually adapt and make improvements. It is almost as if it overcompensates for what may lie ahead. This is how we can slow down the effects of aging.

In a previous section it was concluded that we are all after the best results. While others may tell you that exercise should be fun, that you have to like it, that walking is best . . . I would say this. Fun is an attitude and what is REALLY fun is getting excellent results. Results that you can feel within your muscle fibers and see in the way your clothes fit. We can learn to like what benefits us the most. Don't get me wrong. I don't believe that exercise should be devoid of fun. I do think that people miss out on what may be best for them, though, because they think it doesn't sound "fun". They sweat a little or feel a burn in their muscle and conclude, "this isn't right, I was told this should be fun". Trust me, making *real* progress is quite rewarding, fun, and enjoyable. Think of it this way. If you could make $1000 for 40 hours of sitting at a desk or $1000 for 4 hours of reasonable manual labor with the rest of the week off, which would you choose? A little effort put forth in the right activity pays huge dividends.

Having said that, the proven, single best exercise method to transform body composition from fat to muscle is known *as progressive resistance training*. It is also called strength training, and for most people, includes weight lifting. For the majority of people, strength training has been found to be the most appropriate form of exercise and it provides the greatest amount of health benefits.

Yet strength training is often completely ignored by mainstream authorities, given second fiddle or criticized and mislabeled with age-old myths. Thankfully, this is beginning to change, as more and more people are touting its benefits. Yet much work remains to be done, as approximately 9 out of 10 people are still not aware of the proverbial fountain of youth of strength training. This is regrettable and potentially millions are missing out on some very terrific benefits. Now, let me quickly add, I do not think it is the *only* form of exercise that a person should do. A little further on we will look at other types of exercise and their benefits.

A few years ago, while doing some research, I came across a book called "*Strong Women Stay Young*". This book describes the results of a research experiment at Tufts University School of Nutrition Science and Policy. Tufts was conducting studies, trying to come up with ways to reduce the effects of premature aging and associated chronic diseases. They decided to conduct a strength training experiment, and chose a group of middle-aged women as their test group. Before beginning the experiment, the women's biomarkers were measured. A biomarker is a biological measurement of the human body that determines its "true" biological age (i.e. bone density, blood pressure, strength). For example, if a person is forty years of age and has been taking good care of themselves, their biomarkers may indicate that their body is more similar to that of someone 20 years of age. If they have neglected themselves, their biomarkers may indicate that they are more like someone who is sixty years of age.

After taking their biomarker measurements, the women were placed on a one-year strength-training program. During that year, they were not allowed to change their present eating habits or take part in any other form of exercise. After one year, the women's biomarker measurements were taken again. On average, their measurements had been reduced by 15-20 years! Tufts reported that, "no other program whether diet, medication or aerobic exercise has ever achieved similar results". News spread of this quickly, including to the New England Journal of Medicine. The Keiser Institute of Aging heard of the experiment, and decided to see if similar results could be achieved with senior citizens, both men and women. They conducted a similar study at a nursing home in Boston. The results were even better. Several participants who required walkers and wheelchairs at the time of the experiment were able to walk without assistance after the experiment was over because of their newfound strength.

Strength training benefits the heart as well. Dr. William Winnet, former heart surgeon for over twenty years and the author of *You Can Feel Good All the Time* states, "if everyone in this country would take part in a moderate strength training program, the overall health of our nation would markedly improve." I had an interesting personal experience that illustrates this point. For a period of about 10 years, I did no other form of exercise but intensive weight lifting. Near the end of that time, when I was around 35, I was in my doctor's office getting a physical for a coaching position. The nurse was curious as to what type of physical training program I followed, as my resting heart rate was a 48. She took several measurements and asked, "Do you run marathons or something?" No, I said, "I simply lift weights on a consistent basis". Not to long after that, I read a study by the Weider Institute, which explained why my resting heart rate was so good. Imagine that you are using your bicep muscle to lift a weight. When you do so, the heart sends blood to that working muscle, carrying oxygen and nutrients to the muscle to assist it in completing its task. Those who lift weights, generally train all the major muscle groups of the body week in and week out. As a result, the heart is continually moving blood to working muscles in order to supply oxygen and allow them to complete their work. The heart is also a muscle. Over time, the heart wall begins to thicken and grow stronger. With a thicker and stronger heart wall, the heart is able to "squeeze" more blood into your arteries with each beat. It requires fewer beats and less work to get its job done. Less strain is put on the heart, allowing it to stay healthy and work well for a longer period of time. That explains why my resting heart rate was terrific for my age. You can look forward to the same experience!

Harvard University recently conducted a study solely dedicated to comparing strength training to aerobic exercise to analyze and compare heart health benefits. The study involved 40,000 male doctors. The test group was split in half, with one group using only aerobic exercise and the other strength training. As expected, the aerobic exercisers showed a significant improvement in heart health and a reduction in risk for heart disease. But, the strength trainers showed equal improvement. This was a surprise to those who assumed that the only way to improve cardio-vascular condition was through aerobic effort. A report in the Saturday evening post mirrored the results of that study, and went on to say that strength training may be a more appropriate form of exercise for beginners as it can be easily modified to prevent over exertion while preparing the muscles, bones, joints, ligaments and heart for future aerobic exercise training.

Getting your heart rate up to a certain level and maintaining it for an extended period of time through aerobic exercise is a good idea. Obviously, it helps condition the heart and body and improves overall health. However, it is not an activity that reflects the activities of our lives. How often are you called upon to run for 20 non-stop minutes or climb 25 flights of stairs in a hurry. It could happen, but probably not that often. More likely, you need to be physically able to lift groceries, dig in your garden, trim hedges, or shovel snow. I remember each winter in Pennsylvania, after every heavy snowfall there would be a number of heart attack deaths from people shoveling snow. Shoveling snow is quite demanding, using large muscle groups and brief, yet intense efforts. Strength training, done correctly, is better preparation for shoveling snow (and other everyday activities) than aerobic exercise.

Another objection to strength training is that it will make you stiff, bulky and inflexible. But when done correctly, the exact opposite takes place. Those who train properly become more flexible and operate with greater function. A muscle that is strong and trained through its full range of motion is healthier and more flexible than a weaker, untrained muscle. As a case in point, most readers are probably familiar with Lou Ferrigno, who played, "The Incredible Hulk", and competed as a professional bodybuilder. He won the Mr. Universe competition and also competed against Arnold Schwarzenegger in the movie, "Pumping Iron". During his prime, Lou took part in the old, "Superstars" competition television show. The show brought top performers from nearly every sport to compete against each other in a wide variety of athletic feats. These feats tested their speed, agility, quickness, flexibility, and power. Much to everyone's surprise, Lou Ferrigno, with no other athletic training or background except intensive weight lifting, took second place in the entire competition. Kyle Rote, Jr., a great soccer player, won the competition that year. So much for lack of flexibility and stiffness!

"What about muscular *endurance*? Isn't running a better way to condition the body", many people ask? Yes and no. Aerobics or endurance exercise like running and rowing are all terrific for conditioning the body. It is suggested that you do include an activity of that type in your workout lifestyle eventually. But, aerobics, endurance exercise or "cardio" alone can't provide you with all the benefits of strength training, while strength training can give you the benefits of both. About twenty years ago, an experiment was conducted to test the endurance effects of strength training. At Ball State University, physiologists in the human performance laboratory put a competitive bodybuilder through a series of tests. Mike Katz, a former Mr. USA, took part in a variety of measurements of endurance, aerobic activity, oxygen utilization, etc. Somewhat to their surprise, Mr. Katz' measurements were the best they had ever tested and, in some instances, his results were immeasurable. Granted, Mike Katz was a former pro football player and probably supplemented his workouts with aerobic activity. But clearly, the majority of his training was weight lifting. I have had clients who were unable to perform 10 pushups at the start of their training. After a few months of strength training, they are able to crank out 25-30 pushups with ease.

Hopefully your mind has been opened to the extraordinary benefits of strength training. Perhaps I'm being redundant, but let me stress how especially true this is for women and senior citizens. I will cite a few reasons why this is true in the following chapter where we will briefly examine the more popular types of exercise. As we close this chapter, though, I thought it would be "fitting" to give you a quick run down of how strength training can indeed "lift" your health, energy and spirit to higher and higher planes.

How strength training benefits you!

- Tones your muscles, which looks great and raises your basal metabolism, which causes you to burn more calories 24 hours a day. You'll even burn more calories while you're sleeping!
- Can reverse the natural decline in your metabolism that begins around age 30.
- Energizes you. Energy is developed in muscle cells.
- Assures that you lose fat and hold onto invaluable muscle when "dieting".
- Makes doing all other types of exercise such as aerobics easier and more effective in burning calories.
- Increases the production and release of helpful enzymes and stress fighting hormones.
- Has a positive effect on almost all of your 650+ muscles.
- Slows down the aging clock.
- Decrease body fat.
- Improves flexibility and function of joints, ligaments and muscles.
- Increases aerobic capacity when done correctly.
- Helps us to handle stress better and fortifies the body against stress.
- Prevents and reverses physical frailty.

- Increases insulin sensitivity.
- Decreases your risk of developing adult onset diabetes.
- Relieves symptoms of arthritis.
- Decreases your gastrointestinal transit time, reducing your risk for developing colon cancer.
- Increases blood level of HDL cholesterol (the good type).
- Improves posture.
- Improves the functioning of your immune system.
- Lowers your resting heart rate, a sign of a more efficient, healthy, strong heart.
- Improves your balance and coordination.
- Elevates your mood.
- Can possibly replace hormone therapy.
- Improves the quality of sleep.
- Reduces and lifts depression.
- Helps prevent falls.
- Helps prevent obesity and its many consequences.
- Increases walking speed.
- Increases stair climbing power.
- Can increase overall activity level more than 25%.
- **Resting metabolic rate of strength trainers is on average 15 % higher than non-strength trainers!!!!**
- Seniors can gain strength increases of 113%!
- Improves ability to function with fibromyalgia.
- Strengthens your bones and increases bone density naturally, reducing your risk of developing osteoporosis.
- Improves muscular endurance.
- Develops toned muscles on women . . . NOT big muscles!
- Makes your body stronger and safer for everyday living.
- Builds confidence in your overall approach to life.
- Improves health and function of nerves and nervous system.
- Makes you less prone to low-back injuries.
- Decreases resting blood pressure.

The Keiser Institute states "strength training is safe and effective for all ages, even the very old, and those with chronic conditions such as arthritis, osteoporosis, diabetes, and heart disease". Now you know that strength training can have amazing benefits for virtually any one, from young teen to centenarian. Yes, other forms of exercise offer an extensive array of benefits as well. But no other form of exercise is **as effective nor offers as many benefits** for as *wide a variety* of people.

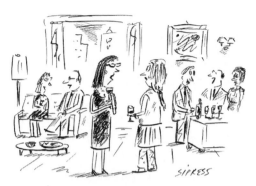

"I don't speak Yoga. I speak Pilates."

Chapter 12

If You Are Hunting Elephants,

Don't Use a BB Gun!

One of the most frequent questions received is, "what do you think of _____ type of exercise?" This chapter is designed to answer those questions. I have been involved in passionate debates over what type of exercise is best. In the fitness magazines, you will find "fitness wars" going on as each advocate vehemently vouches for the validity and value of their personal favorite. While understandable, the result of this bickering can leave readers confused and disillusioned. The following information will help to put things in perspective.

First of all, any form of exercise is certainly better than doing nothing. All exercise can and will produce some of the benefits I ascribe to strength training. The important thing with any method of exercise is to do it correctly and consistently. If you are currently exercising on a consistent basis, congratulations! If you have a particular exercise that you look forward to and benefit from, further congratulations. I certainly do not want to confuse you or discourage you from positive efforts and activities.

But it has been my experience that people will contact me with a question and when I ask them if they are strength training, they often reply, "no, I'm doing such and such". My usual response is to encourage them to continue doing such and such, but to a lesser degree, making room to implement a progressive resistance program as well. To reach their healthiness goals, they need to have the right ammo and the best weapon. Sometimes, dabbling in the latest fad exercise craze takes us away from our primary goal and makes it harder to hit the mark. It is like trying to hunt down an elephant with a bb gun. That wouldn't get us many elephants!

Some of these distractions might include popular forms of exercise like running/jogging, treadmills, swimming, pilates, yoga, tai chi, bodyweight exercises, tai bo, walking, spinning, and aerobics classes. When evaluating these options, consider how effective they are at transforming body composition and reducing excess body fat. That is the primary goal (our elephant) and, when accomplished, will bring a bounty of health and fitness benefits.

Of course, each of these forms of exercise can have a place in a healthiness lifestyle. In fact, I recommend advancing trainees develop a fitness triangle, each side representing a different activity and function of exercise. Ideally, the three sides of the triangle are strength training (weight lifting), endurance exercise, and aerobic/cardiovascular exercises. Many people, though, don't initially have time for all three but still want maximum benefit from their efforts. Strength training is their answer. It can provide substantial aerobic and flexibility benefits while building the miracle of muscle. If you find yourself having to choose between the 3 types of activities, choose strength training.

If you have developed a consistent program of strength training and are interested in developing the other two sides of the triangle, there is much to choose from. Pilates, yoga, tai chi, body weight exercises and swimming are endurance activities that are currently popular. Treadmills, tai bo, jogging, running, aerobic classes, and spinning, are examples of effective aerobic/cardiovascular exercise. A recommended goal for those who wish to do all 3 types of exercise would be to spend their time as follows: 42% strength building (weights lifting), 32% endurance exercise (body weight exercises), 29% aerobic activities (walking, jogging, sprinting).

The majority of time *initially* however, is spent weight training, followed by a brief stint of moderate aerobic activity. This routine, coupled with improved eating patterns, allows for rapid improvements in fitness and overall health. As strength, body fat levels and aerobic capacity improve to superior standards, aerobic intensity is increased, and more endurance type activities can be added to the program such as body weight movements, calisthenics, and so on. This "formula" is always a little different, as each person is unique, and their unique plan will require modifications. But one pattern is almost certain. Everyone should improve their overall strength (via weight training) before they engage in the other exercise activities, in order to safeguard their health and avoid injury. Many health/fitness experts suggest that the average person spend up to six weeks in weight lifting, especially for the lower body, before taking up jogging or running. Overuse injuries amongst runners has been found to occur in over 75% of people within the first year. Strengthening and enhancing muscles, bones, and joints beforehand, could have prevented some of these injuries. Yoga, which seems relatively safe, is also experiencing the same phenomenon. Yoga injuries have been occurring in increasing numbers, as deconditioned individuals are attempting yoga exercises beyond their strength levels. Most individuals would be wise to strengthen themselves through weight training first or at least simultaneously with other fitness endeavors.

Chapter 13

Fad Fitness . . . . What's In, What's Out?

The fitness business, like other areas of life, is not immune to fads. It is important to spend a moment addressing this, and the implications it has for the average person seeking improved healthiness. Many people turn to the latest literature or their local health club for assistance. Fitness magazines, products and health clubs are lucrative and competitive. Ironically, health clubs are usually supported by around 10% of a community's population. Keeping and adding members is their challenge, and in an effort to do that, they must market, and keep things interesting. In an attempt to keep and attract members, the fitness industry is continually looking for ways to make their "product" more appealing, as it seems we humans need constant stimulation and the masses of people see exercise and fitness as boring and unappealing. But here again, is the problem. Many of these fitness "discoveries" are promoted by the those who are usually practicing fitness already, are more fit than average, enjoy exercise, and are looking for new ways to challenge themselves. They find a new way to challenge themselves and, suddenly, a new exercise "movement" is born. Exercise "junkies" run to it, embrace it, and in due time, it is proclaimed as the savior of the unfit. Almost immediately, the infomercials start cranking, expelling the miraculous qualities of an ancient fitness method comprised of long kept secrets and promoted by a mysterious health guru, but now available to everyone.

What is the problem with that, you may ask? Here is the problem. There is no "magic" in a name. For example, pilates, tai bo, tai chi and yoga have become somewhat vogue in the past decade. Sometimes it seems their appeal is in their fancy sounding foreign flair and celebrity endorsements. *PLEASE* realize, all of these activities can be great forms of exercise. But much of what you will read and hear advertised is untrue and sometimes suggests a fitness "rose garden" to a person currently wallowing in a wellness weed patch. The promoters of these programs are often *not* giving people true foundational knowledge of how their bodies work (physiology) and how to improve them. Far worse, several offer themselves as the *exclusive* solution while criticizing and contributing to outright falsehoods and myths about other types of exercise.

Several of these disciplines are especially critical of weight lifting, saying that it will give you "big bulky stiff muscles, injure you, yada, yada, yada. Then, some make claims for themselves that are misleading and **physiologically impossible**. Pilates, for example, makes claims it can give you a "lean dancers body" and "longer muscles". Others propose that their exercise method will help to fill your mind, spirit and soul with inner peace. Think I'm kidding? Read the books and listen to the advertisements. The truth is that often times their marketing methods are simply designed to position them as the one and only best method, which of course leads back to the insatiable quest of the almighty dollar$. Yes, you can injure yourself lifting weights, as you can with yoga, tai bo, wobble boards, aerobics, jogging, or virtually any activity. Driving your car into oncoming traffic will probably kill you too. Does that mean we should not drive? Of course not, that's why we have driver's training. Learn, progress gradually and follow the correct methods in most disciplines (including weight lifting/strength training) and you will be fine.

Don't be fooled by the magical sound of a name or method. Just because a practice sounds alluring or trendy does not mean it is any more effective than an ordinary method. The responsible thing to do is teach a person how their body truly works, and show them how to improve it based upon proven results and science. Telling a person that they can get a "dancers body" through a specific exercise movement is misleading. Having people climb on wobble boards before they have foundational balance makes little sense, except perhaps to the person selling the wobble boards!

As you will see, the message will be consistent. You will not be told that you should avoid all other types of exercise or that another exercise type is all wrong and totally lame. Rather, the message is to use what is *best*, not just what everyone else is doing because it is the latest and greatest "hot" thing. You will be encouraged to use what works, using a variety of methods with strength training/ weight lifting as the foundation, combined with any other activities that promote success.

Again, if you enjoy an activity and its fun for you, continue in it. But ask yourself if it is the best alternative available to you for reaching your primary goals? As you consider your options, we will briefly evaluate the strengths and weakness of various exercise choices. Many of these have been with us throughout history; others were developed in the last century while some have become "all the rage" in the late 1990's and early 2000's.

Walking

My family and I enjoy going for walks in the neighborhood. Nearly every night, and sometimes morning as well, we take a stroll trough the neighborhood. It is relaxing, great to smell the fresh air, see the birds and talk to neighbors. There is also a steep hill in our neighborhood that is not an easy task to walk up and we usually include that for fitness fun. Walking is definitely good for you, physically, mentally, and emotionally. But it is NOT the best exercise. Remember our previous definitions of exercise? Words like *make an inroad* and *mess up your physiology* were used in order to communicate that the best forms of exercise are those that require our body to perform a task greater than what it is used to. Most of us have been walking our entire lives and while we should walk more often, it does not really challenge the upper half of our body very well. It makes little "inroad" overall and requires little adaptation by the body. If you are currently walking on a regular basis, keep going. But, you ought to keep records, timing yourself and challenging yourself to walk a little further in less time, and including more uphill climbing when feasible. And in addition to walking, I would emphatically encourage (even beg!) you to include the other workouts in this book.

Pilates and Yoga

A gentleman named Joseph Pilates developed "Pilates". He originally called his particular method "Contrology" because its intent was to help us develop better control of our body. He was definitely a fitness pioneer, and developed several inventions and contraptions to implement his methods. Today, a variety of machines are sold for a few thousand dollars to perform pilates methods. The techniques can help you improve the flexibility and endurance of the body. It has limited ability to build muscle and improve strength. The fancy machines are not all bad, but they are not needed to do many of the basic pilates exercises. If you have access to one and instruction on how to properly use it, terrific. Pilates and yoga can be beneficial for most of us. Do realize though, they can also be difficult and challenging, especially for beginners. If you want to pursue these activities, slowly progress into them, learn the correct techniques and weight lift on alternating days.

Personally, I do not take part in what most would call pilates or yoga, but do perform about 15-20 minutes of body weight exercises on my non-weight lifting days. These body weight exercises have in many cases been practiced in health and fitness routines throughout the 18th and 19th century. I will include examples of the bodyweight exercises I perform in the workout section of this book.

Be aware, despite claims to the contrary, pilates *cannot* lengthen your muscles. Muscle length is a genetic trait, which we cannot change. Gifted athletes have uncommon muscle lengths that contribute to some of the unique feats they are able to perform. This "muscle lengthening" marketing and "dancer body" nonsense are falsehoods promoted by some pilates entrepreneurs. In reality, all of us can improve and change the way our bodies look. By losing excess body fat, adding muscle and strengthening bone, we can make very noticeable improvements and get closer to reaching our genetic potential. My daughter, who is 9 years old, has what most would call a dancers body. She is tall, slender and graceful on the dance floor. However, she would be tall and slender even if she never danced! The fact that she is graceful on the dance floor comes from a few years of dedicated practice. This "dancers body" premise is similar to the one sold to the naturally skinny kid. He is told that he can look like the massive muscled bodybuilder in the advertisements if he just uses the miracle supplement they feature. He buys all of the miracle supplements, performs the workouts in the muscle magazines and is then disappointed. False promises not only rip people off but also discourage them and lead to feelings of failure, which is the exact opposite of what most of us need.

Honest and professional pilates practitioners and promoters will tell you that pilates alone is not effective at reducing excess body fat. They will stress that it primarily helps to improve balance and flexibility. But doesn't it seem silly to spend time working on improving flexibility when a person has a dangerously high percentage of body fat and very little muscle on their body? They are simply going through the inane activity of making their fat more flexible?

People should be told the truth. The focus should be on lifelong health, vitality and vigor, with an improved overall appearance as a side benefit. Pilates can help to improve your health, fitness and wellness. The idea that you will become lithe and lean **through it and it alone** while strength training will cause you to stiffen and bulk up is bunk. Yes, there are some bulked-up and stiff looking bodybuilders. But they are only a *tiny fraction* of those who strength train and most have worked at an almost superhuman level to achieve those results. That is most likely not your goal. Hopefully, your goal is to become a lean, fat-incinerating, anti-aging, wellness machine!

There is another other thing that is interesting. Pilates and yoga books feature many age-old stretching and callisthenic exercises that have been practiced in athletics and gym classes for decades. Now, they appear in these books with names I can't pronounce or understand half the time (like Dhanurasana?). What makes a crunch a "yoga crunch"? They are the same crunches we have all loved and endured forever.

Core Training

Core training is a phrase that has been recently introduced into the world of fitness. The idea behind core training is that exercising the "core" of the body should be a key priority of any fitness routine. The core consists primarily of the abdominal region, lower back and spine, buttocks, hips, and upper legs. The theory is that this is the center of the body where many poor health issues of the body occur. It is well known that this is the origin of power and strength on the human body, and thus it makes sense to focus much of our effort on improving in these areas.

Pilates, yoga, aerobics and some "functional" strength training classes often use the term core training in describing their methods. Core training is a smart idea, and needs to be done in any exercise method. But it is nothing new, even though we hear the word used often these days. Part of core training emphasized is "balance" training as well. What seems ironic is that both traditional weight lifting and body weight calisthenics have always emphasized, developed and strengthen the core. They just didn't coin the term.

Burpees, one of my favorites from elementary gym class, will work your core as well as any new fangled wobble boards or ancient exercise practices. Some of the mainstay exercises of weight lifting, such as lunges, squats, abdominal crunches, one-arm rows, will work our core as well or better than any exercise method. For decades weight training was labeled as "unsafe", partially because people might lose their balance. Now, all kind of contraptions have hit the scene that require people to stand on boards and balls while exercising to improve their balance, stability, and "core".

Meanwhile, weight lifting is incorrectly dubbed as not being a "full body exercise". Stability, balance and core strength are enhanced when one develops a well-muscled, lean and trained body. One of the best ways to build such a body, as millions have done, is through traditional weight training, proper eating and sleep. Also, the principles of physiology are largely ignored when one makes such a statement. Take bicep curls for example. Whether they are performed standing or sitting, it is not simply the biceps that are being worked. The entire cardiovascular, respiratory and nervous system is involved. In addition, many of the stabilizer muscles of the "core" help to hold the body in place. No doubt though, you should include other exercises of the primary muscle groups, such as your chest, upper back and hips to stimulate your entire body. Performing your strength training with dumbbells and using alternating or single arm/leg movements will help to involve the "core" of your body to a greater degree, and several of the exercises in this book are demonstrated in this fashion. But make no mistake; to develop the core, standard weight training may be all it takes.

Michael Yessis, Ph.D., a professor at California State University, Fullerton and researcher in kinesiology and exercise technique stated that free weight exercise develops balance (especially core muscle strength) more effectively than the use of balance equipment. In fact he calls the current focus on core training, "wobbly logic" in that many of these newer techniques may be less safe and effective in setting out to accomplish what weight training already does.

Aerobics, Spinning, Tai Bo

Aerobics activities that move large muscle groups for an extended period of time at various intensities contribute to improved heart, lung and overall body health. They also contribute to fat loss when done correctly. However, perhaps the greatest benefit of aerobic and cardiovascular exercise is that it creates additional, "pathways" to working muscles, thereby allowing for enhanced oxygen uptake in the muscles. Thus, muscles can perform their function more easily, which reduces the amount of strain and effort required of the heart. However, aerobic activity does not impact body composition as much as some would lead you to believe. The body composition of some aerobics instructors, in fact, is not within the desired range. "Skinny fat" aerobics instructor syndrome comes about from doing excessive aerobics with no strength training. **Excessive aerobics can cause the same effect as incorrect dieting, that is, it can cause muscle loss.**

Many aerobics, spinning and tai bo classes last up to one hour. This is not needed, and can actually cause you to regress and miss your goals. The best way to perform aerobic activity is immediately after strength training, for 12-15 minutes, at the highest intensity possible, within your target heart range. If a person wants to perform aerobics on their non-weight/strength training days, they can do so for up to 20 minutes, but longer is not better. Unless you are training for a marathon or triathlon, twenty minutes is enough to get the health benefits, burn fat and preserve muscle. Most people do not need to worry about doing aerobic exercise on their non-strength training days at first though. Instead, they should focus their efforts on the weight lifting, followed by brief and intense aerobic activity, eat correctly and rest on their "off" days, until they have added enough muscle and shed enough fat that their abdominal muscles are visible. At that point they may be able to progress to aerobics on off days.

The unfortunate thing is this. Most people do the opposite of this, which is a mistake and why they get poor results. Usually when I go to the gym early in the morning, I walk past all the treadmills and see them largely occupied by middle-aged men with big bellies and women who are overweight. They are usually on the treadmill when I get to the gym and **still** on it when I leave 30-35 minutes later! Meanwhile, I will have gone into the free weight room, which is usually not crowded except for a few fitter and leaner looking men and women. It always strikes me that the fittest people are in the weight room and the least fit people are on the treadmills. The unfit people are using the wrong tools, at least when it comes to time and effort applied in pursuit of their healthiness goals.

By building muscle **first** and using the treadmill **after,** they would get two benefits. First, as they add muscle, the amount of calories they will burn all day long increases. With that added muscle, the amount of calories they burn will go up even further as they do their aerobic work. Many have got it backwards. Fitness experts agree that the most common mistake made in the gym is not performing strength training.

Another way to look at it is this, when you spend twenty minutes on the treadmill, you are burning calories, but the moment you step foot off of the treadmill, much of the elevated calorie burning stops almost immediately. An intense twenty minutes with the weights however, keeps you burning calories for at least the next four hours and, with increases in muscle, for as long as 24 hours. To take advantage of this fact, people are far better off to perform their aerobics immediately after weight training when metabolism is nearly peaked. By doing so, they can drive their fat burning potential through the roof and save bucket loads of time as well.

So, do your aerobics. But do them AFTER weight training and for no longer than fifteen minutes. Follow this up by eating well, sleeping enough and you will soon be looking and felling swell.

Isometrics

Isometrics were quite popular back in the 60's. It is a form of strength training where the resistance does not move, and where the muscle length does not change. This particular type of exercise can be beneficial, but in my opinion, is really for the more advanced exerciser. Astronauts and soldiers are taught this method, because of the confines in which they sometimes must live. A person with no other options for movement could use this form of exercise, for example, by pushing down on one hand while resisting upwards with the other hand. That would serve to stimulate the muscles and joints of the arm and shoulder regions. In the case of a prisoner of war or someone who has no other options available, isometrics are perhaps the only way to go.

I use isometric principles when I hang from a parallel bar. I grasp the bar with my hands and hang at full length, timing myself, several days a week. I find this to be a great way to stretch my spine and entire upper body, while strengthening my grip. The goal is to continually increase my "hang time". There are other ways to apply this principle, such as doing handstands for time, etc. As a teenager, though, I spent almost a year trying to build muscle and strength strictly with isometric exercise and calisthenics. The results were barely apparent, although I am sure it was better than doing nothing. Once I took up weight training, though, my results skyrocketed.

Jogging/Running

When "aerobic" exercise, popularized by Dr. Kenneth Cooper, became the fitness movement in America, the practice of jogging literally took off. Millions of people took up jogging and running as their primary fitness activity. Overall, the health of our nation improved, and heart attack numbers declined. The future was looking fitter. But, like a diet done wrong, the results did not last long. Because most of the joggers and runners were not building muscle at the same time, many joggers actually jogged off some of their muscle and became fatter people with slower metabolisms. Many took up jogging who were weak, especially throughout their lower bodies. Overuse injuries began to occur. I have talked with many former joggers and runners, who enjoyed the activity but are no longer able to partake in it due to injury and chronic pain in the knees, ankles and hip joints. This is unfortunate because jogging and running are positive activities that most of us could and should try to benefit from.

If those jogging had combined it with strength training, things would have been better. Many of the injuries could have been avoided. Also unfortunate is that while heart attack deaths have declined, the number of heart attacks overall have increased. Dr. Cooper has since learned of the missing, "strength" link, and now promotes that as well, much to his credit. His Cooper Clinic and fitness books now include weight lifting and he recently stated, "You should change your focus on exercise as you age. You need to save those joints, concentrate more on building muscle, and less on aerobics".

Strength training should begin (under supervision) in our teens. Our society is SO sedentary, compared to even fifty years ago. The bodies of our entire population have become soft, weak, and unchallenged. Do not wait until you are older and starting to become feeble to get strong. I started weight training at 14. It is now thirty plus years later and I am still at it. I know there are thousands like me who can say the same thing. My sixteen-year-old son started strength training seriously at 15. He has become much leaner, stronger, fitter and more muscular rather quickly.

Personally, I use jogging/running as my favorite aerobic exercise. I find nothing more challenging, effective and invigorating as a good jog/run. Nevertheless, I sometimes do not have a lot of enthusiasm about going for a jog. But knowing it will challenge my heart, lungs, legs and spirit, off I go anyway, putting one foot in front of the other. Eventually, I start to enjoy the process, and by the time I am done, I am invigorated. I should add, I run with confidence, knowing that I have prepared myself to run. My lower body and heart have been adequately strengthened to handle the rigors of jogging. Others agree that it is wise to build strength first before attempting to jog/run. Don Chu, a respected health and fitness professor, states that one should spend at least six weeks in a strength training program before starting to jog. I want to stress again, that in order to realize the greatest benefit and avoid overuse injuries, a jog/run should be brief. An average of 12-20 minutes after strength training will be adequate. As your fitness improves, you can simply go a little faster during this time. If you are not yet in condition to jog/run, simply walk as fast as you can. A good way to progress from walking to jogging is to occasionally jog 20-30 yards throughout your walk, increasing the distance a little each session until eventually you are jogging the entire time. That way you will be more likely to be able to enjoy the benefits of jogging/running late into your active life.

Swimming

Swimming is a great form of exercise and has benefited people for centuries. It is a good all around body conditioner, improving strength, endurance, and aerobic capacity and is refreshing and relaxing as well. Swimming seems to be helpful with those with arthritis, and water aerobics and exercise are quite popular with many people. Several of my clients have participated in swimming or water activities as an adjunct to their strength training, and you have probably guessed that I would recommend you do the same. Swimming can provide benefits that other exercise can't duplicate because of the fact it is based in the water. That same factor somewhat limits its benefits as well, however. In short, we don't spend all of our time in the water. We spend much of it on land. Thus, we need to spend some time in "land training" as well. And remember, swimming alone will not accomplish the transformation that water and weights combined can. Arthritis and joint pain are improved as we add muscle to our frames. Swimming *alone* is not the most effective way to preserve or add muscle. Muscle makes doing everything easier and relieves pressure off of the rest of the body.

Some of you may remember Jack Lalanne, the famous fitness pioneer. He reportedly swims up to 1 hour a day. Most of us do not have that kind of time available, but could enjoy swimming benefits with a short swim a few days each week. Jack Lalanne also lifts weights for one hour *BEFORE* he engages in swimming! Work strength training into your fitness program along with your swimming. As you do, I am confident you will be pleased at how much easier everyday activities become (including swimming) in addition to the other health and appearance benefits.

Tai Chi

Tai Chi originates from the martial arts. Recently I began to study it a little and so far, this is what I see: tai chi, like all forms of exercise, is far better than doing nothing. But, it is a slow moving and softer exercise method and will have little impact on your body composition. It has been promoted as being a good way to help with arthritis suffers and for senior citizens to get moving. Tai Chi, however, does also include and promote a spiritual element of "centering", which I think is a little weird and not the purpose of exercise, at least in my training and experience. If you desire to utilize tai chi, I recommend you do it on your non-strength training days. It will help to improve your flexibility, balance, muscle endurance and body control. Those are all good things. Whether it can align you with the moon and stars is still yet to be derived, but I wouldn't hold my breath.

Bodyweight Exercises/Calisthenics

Bodyweight exercises (a.k.a. BWE) are something most of us are familiar with. These include good old pushups, sit-ups, pull-ups and so on. In this day of high technology and thousand dollar exercise machines, BWE are one of the most overlooked methods to improving health. Wait a minute, you say, what about strength training? Weight lifting and conventional body weight exercises/calisthenics are the forgotten foundations of health and fitness. But make no mistake, when it comes to improving most of the measurements of fitness and health, body weight exercises run a close second to strength training. Admittedly, I have not always felt this way. I spent my first year and a half as a teenager doing strictly bodyweight and isometric exercises in pursuit of my goals to build muscle, strength, and health. At the time, I was too weak to do very many pull-ups, but was able to do a few pushups, burpees, sit-ups and so forth. The progress I saw was barely noticeable to the naked eye.

However, a few years later I began to lift weights, and almost immediately I began to see and feel muscles that I didn't realize I possessed. When it comes to the science of *adding* significant muscle, weight lifting is more effective than body weight exercises alone. Now that I have increased my strength and added some muscle through weight lifting, I find BWE to be a terrific supplement to my workouts.

The benefits of BWE's are that they require no equipment, can be done anywhere and anytime, can be done throughout your lifetime, and will improve your total body strength, flexibility, cardiovascular health, and endurance. Their greatest benefit may be in building muscular endurance and overall body stamina. There is nothing that awakens the body like a good set of calisthenics. BWE give more hustle to your muscle. For example, the heart gets pumping powerfully and rather quickly in a set of body weight squats. In fact, BWE's can be quite challenging and downright hard. Initially, most of them are beyond the scope and capability of beginners or those who are out of shape. The truth is, I think many of us have avoided these standard exercises because we know how strenuous they actually are. We are more willing to take on less challenging activities like yoga, pilates and tai chi. BWE's are difficult for most of us at first because we have lost much of the muscle we once owned. As you add muscle through weight lifting, go back to your childhood friends of pushups, back bridges and so on. Progress a little each week, and you will soon be feeling like the stud or studette you perhaps were or dreamed of being in high school!

I don't agree with the trainers who say that weight training should be dropped altogether in favor of body weight exercises. There are not many who say this, but there are a few. Their argument is that weight-training can causes injuries, does not provide the endurance benefits, and requires equipment or a gym. Some of their arguments hold a little water, but others do not. Many of the current advocates and students of BWE **only**, are younger males, with a few hardliner middle age males like myself who enjoy challenging themselves physically. Most of the BWE only promoters I have seen have already been exercising in a disciplined fashion for decades. I believe that the rest of the population could benefit from BWE's but everyone should start with a moderate strength/weight-lifting program.

One final thought on BWE's. The Navy Seals, all military branches, and many Olympic athletes focus heavily on basic calisthenics and weight lifting to finely tune their bodies. They don't rely solely on pilates, yoga or any "mind body" connection concoctions. Forcing your body to push itself harder and harder with basic BWE will involve plenty of "mind body" connection and mental toughness!

Examples of body weight exercises I use are demonstrated in the work out section and are those exercises that do not include weights. These exercises can be done on both weight training and non-weight training days if desired. The reason being that they do not make the same "inroad" into your muscle fibers as weight lifting does. Thus, BWE do not require as much recuperation time as weight lifting does.

Hydraulic Resistance Programs
Over the past few years, several gym chains have been springing up around the country which feature hydraulic resistance equipment. The better known of these include "Curves" and "Slender Lady".

These gyms are quite popular. Curves was the fastest growing franchise in the country when it first started. A question that I receive at many conferences is, "What do you think of Curves?" The response to that question is this. First of all, Curves utilizes hydraulic resistance equipment for a significant part of their program. Hydraulic resistance is a form of strength training similar to weight lifting. As such, Curves can be a good thing. They have done a terrific job of introducing many women to the benefits of strength training in a supportive, encouraging, and educational environment. In truth, I wish I had thought of the concept.

The real question, though, is whether this type of equipment is as effective as free weights or standard weight machines. Exercise physiologists consistently state that "resistance is resistance" to the human body. Our muscles cannot tell whether the resistance is coming from a dumbbell, weight machine, or hydraulic equipment. The Keiser Company, which manufactures high quality hydraulic equipment has conducted experiments from high-level athletes to senior citizens, and proven its effectiveness in adding strength and muscle. I have personally worked out with Keiser's equipment and found the workout capable of making an "inroad" comparable to other forms of resistance.

The results with Curves, and similar companies, speak for themselves. Thousands of women have been able to add muscle, shed excess body fat, improve their overall health and become consistent exercisers as a result of their services. Another valuable aspect is that they conduct nutrition education geared towards maximizing results through their exercise programs. I am not thoroughly knowledgeable of their nutrition curriculum, but do know that it emphasizes increased protein, reduction of processed carbohydrates, increased consumption of vegetables and moderate healthy fat intake.

There is really only one drawback to the hydraulic circuit training gyms. Many of those who become members at these facilities are new exercisers and show significant improvements initially. The body is quite adaptive though, and in order to continue progressing and making improvements, one must continually challenge the body and force it to adapt. This can be done in a number of ways. Increasing the amount of weight, length of workouts, speed of movement, or type of resistance. Some trainers have theorized that those who exercise solely on hydraulic equipment may be missing out on **all** of the improvements they could see by also utilizing free weights, and standard weight machines. I have had the same thought, and know from personal experience that a workout I have been performing can begin to feel comfortable, but by changing the type of resistance/exercise slightly, can become quite challenging again.

Dr. Wayne Westcott performed an experiment to test this hypothesis. He took a group of women who had been exercising on hydraulic only equipment and placed them on a new routine, using standard weight machines, with a similar type of circuit training routine. Before the experiment began, body fat, strength, and similar measurements were taken. After six weeks, measurements were again taken, and every single woman in the group showed marked improvement in body fat, strength and their health and fitness levels.

So the advice is simply this. If you are currently involved in a hydraulics only strength routine, realize that you would likely get some additional improvements by adding free weight or standard weight equipment exercises. They will not make you, "all buffed up" or manly looking, despite the marketing myths and stone-age thinking that persists.

Chapter 14

The Strength of the Argument

*"I live temperately, drink little wine, and do daily exercise
with the dumbbell."*

Benjamin Franklin

The fitness lifestyle recommended for most people has been thoroughly discussed. Three types of exercise would become part of their routine. As you may recall, these three types include strength training, bodyweight/endurance exercises, and cardiovascular training. You will achieve a good level of fitness with just one type, a better level of fitness by utilizing two types, and **THE BEST** level of fitness by using all three.

Before we wrap this chapter up and finally get into our actual workout, a final plea for strength training/weight training must be made. Why? Because I just returned from a conference where I met two different individuals who NEED the benefits of strength training in their lives. Yet, their doctors, through lack of expertise and ignorance of strength training, are not helping their patients get what is best for them. This is very frustrating. Patients are getting less than the best treatment from doctors who may be very knowledgeable and fine doctors, but who seem to be quite ignorant of how to promote REAL health, fitness and wellness without the use of drugs, surgery or inferior fitness routines.

One gentleman I met at the conference had suffered a heart attack several years earlier. To his credit, he has been following doctors' orders and running on a treadmill 6 days per week. His doctor had told him that he should try to get his heart rate into his target zone in order to improve health and fitness. Unfortunately, this routine, while of some benefit, is shortchanging this mans progress. The gentleman explained to me that he has a nagging shoulder injury, and a sore upper thigh muscle that he inadvertently pulled while simply lifting his leg. When he participated in a light calisthenics class with me, he struggled to do basic exercises and stretches. He could not do one complete pushup and was unable to perform 10 body weight squats. The exercise program this doctor has given him is *substandard*, and leaving him weak and at risk for both injury and illness. This man could drastically improve his health by taking up strength training.

Another woman I met there was telling me how discouraged she was because her doctor had just told her to *quit* lifting weights. It seems she has fibromyalgia, and he felt that the "high impact" of weight lifting was making her condition worse. Apparently, her doctor knows nothing about strength training and I dare say has done little research on fibromyalgia and the benefits of strength training for that condition.

The woman told me that her current exercise routine consisted of about 40 minutes of "cardio" followed by 20 minutes of strength training. You know by now that she has it all backwards. She should be doing the exact opposite, and for shorter periods of time. And I have no doubt that it was the cardio that was too high impact and caused the flair up in her muscles. A study from Harvard Medical School suggests the use of ADDING strength training to the regimen of a person suffering from fibromyalgia, not removing it. The lady in question should seriously consider finding a more knowledgeable and ambitious doctor.

Suppose you went to the hospital and found out that another patient received better treatment than you did because they were a relative of the doctors or a prominent citizen in the community? I imagine that you would be a little upset. So would most of us. It seems ironic to me that professional athletes, Olympic athletes, and our fighting forces almost all use weight lifting to condition, and when necessary, rehab their bodies. They also use calisthenics and some form of running. Yes, they use other forms of training as well. But I believe it is safe to say that these three activities form the core of their physical work. Their goal, of course, is to be in action, at the highest level, as quickly as possible. They expect, demand and utilize nothing but the best methods. So why do we, average, everyday folks, accept and use less than the best methods for conditioning, and then wonder why we get less than the best results?

This seems to be especially true of women. I have read studies saying that, on average, women receive inferior medical treatment than men. That of course is uncool and unacceptable. It makes me wonder, then, why so many women seem to voluntarily accept less than the best methods available to improve their fitness and health. Perhaps I am wrong, but I don't think so. So my challenge would be this. Take a look at the highest-level athletic competitors in the world, both male and female. Find out what their training systems consist of. I am confident that you will find it is **not** based on one method, and that it will *include* more aggressive, active and assertive methods than most of the currently popular mind-body, centering practices proliferating in health clubs around the country. I am also sure you will find that it involves strength training. What if you don't want to be high-level you ask? Obviously, you may not be trying for a Gold medal, but wouldn't we at least want to reach our highest level? What other level makes sense, I ask? To achieve the best, it seems senseless to use less than the best methods.

Calorie burning always seems to be a concern of exercisers. Many of us have seen the graphs of activities accompanied by the amount of calories each burns. Most of the standard physical activities are usually included such as walking, swimming, aerobics class, etc. Sometimes even normal everyday activates such as sweeping the floor or vacuuming are listed. Occasionally, "weight lifting" shows up, but not often. When weight lifting does show up, a very low amount of calories burned is given. This is misleading and, unfortunately, they are leaving out key information that would be helpful. First of all, they use an "average" person to make these determinations. Is this average person male or female? What is their body type? How much do they weigh and what percentage of their weight is fat? You see, two people can weigh 180 lbs. and one could have 10 more pounds of muscle on their body than the other. The one with more muscle, burns far more calories doing ANYTHING, even sitting on the couch! Also, these charts may say that swimming three days a week for twenty minutes will burn so and so amount of calories. Good information. But what the chart doesn't say is that by adding only 5 pounds of muscle to your body, you could burn an additional 250-450 calories per day (1750-3150 week) without doing *any activity*. And, the best way to get that muscle is with weight lifting.

Even some of America's earliest and greatest leaders and achievers took advantage of the awesome benefits of weight lifting. These wise and gifted individuals evidently understood the dynamics of how to achieve the highest levels of fitness. In their quest to lead extraordinary lives of service and contribution, they utilized strength training as a tool to be prepared, ready and steady. Theodore Roosevelt credits much of his poor health turnaround and resulting robustness to his strength training pursuits. Before Teddy, one of the wisest Americans ever, Ben Franklin, utilized weight lifting in his daily health regimen. It could be argued that Ben Franklin was the first "Wellness" pioneer in America. His innate wisdom led to the development of the Farmers Almanac and the tried and true, "early to bed, early to rise, makes a man healthy, wealthy, and wise." We too, would be wise to exercise daily, and include a little weight lifting along the way. Unlike so many 'new" methods, weight lifting is not a fad and it has stood the test of time. Yoga often claims that it has been practiced for 2000 years. Strength training can make the same claim in that it began with a wrestler named Milo, 250 B.C. Milo was the wrestler who discovered that the fine art of lifting a small calf everyday. His strength grew in proportion to the growth of the calf. We are able to do the same, but our forms of resistance are a little easier to handle!

Youth/Teenagers

As of this writing, one of the most prevalent topics in the media is childhood obesity. I have probably attended at least 50 meetings on this topic. Unfortunately, none of the meetings attended ever really accomplish much. Most of the meetings are conducted by a wide variety of "experts" who proclaim various solutions to reducing obesity in our youth. What always strikes me as interesting, however, is that so many of the adults in attendance at these meetings are themselves not in shape! Very few of them are consistent exercisers, many lack knowledge of the physiology of leanness, and rarely have any of them ever helped another individual become fit.

Having read this far, you now have more understanding about these things than 99 out of 100 people in this country. So you won't be surprised to learn that one of the big factors creating obesity in our youth is the lack of muscle on their bodies. We could help them immensely by providing age-appropriate strength training programs. This topic is not without controversy, but enough evidence is in to support the claim. Wayne Wescott, along with many others, has written several research articles and books demonstrating these findings. The exercises outlined in this book can be used to improve the fitness of your children as well. For those under the age of thirteen, it is recommend using weights that can be lifted slowly and smoothly for at least 15 repetitions. This way, safety of joints and ligaments will be assured, yet stimulation of muscle and bone growth will be enhanced.

Several body weight only exercises are included in this book as well and these can help your child get moving in the right direction. Like adults, the use of resistance training to improve the fitness of kids is largely overlooked and misunderstood. If a young person is ever going to shed excess fat and improve their fitness levels, they will need to add more muscle. This, in turn, will crank up their metabolism. Strength training truly gives the overweight kids a chance to excel, build confidence and self-esteem. Rather than being humiliated and red faced because they are last in a race or unable to perform a pull-up, they can outperform everyone else. As a larger child adds muscle to their body, performing all other activities requires less effort, and the possibility of them becoming more active increases with their added strength, muscle and confidence. For those children who are struggling with obesity, strength training with resistance may be the most appropriate form of exercise. This is especially true for significantly obese kids.

Think of a large overweight child struggling to keep up with other kids running around a track or trying to do a sit-up or pushup. Rather than have a positive affect, the opposite is usually true. Highlighting their weaknesses, rather than their strengths, could further damage self-image and confidence. However, larger kids actually do well and experience success when they strength train. In fact, they can often lift more than their peer, which encourages them to continue exercising. Many of these kids are endomorphs (thick boned, large framed people) and are labeled obese using the body mass index formulas. The truth is they may not be obese; they might just be large people. Regardless, the larger kids are generally stronger than their smaller counterpoints. Because they are stronger, they can benefit from strength training perhaps more than any other exercise type.

It is just not, "larger" children who can benefit though. Body image and self-confidence are serious issues for many young people, despite whatever size they may be. I remember reading several years back of a study about young people and different types of exercise. The study found that strength training with weights, for both males and females, received the highest scores in self-reported improvements in confidence and body image.

The Fitness Formula

The *best* way to reach your health and fitness goals, will be to include three types of exercise. That includes strength training with resistance (usually weights), body weight endurance exercises, and brief periods (10-20 minutes) of cardiovascular exercise. In the next chapter we will begin to construct your workout.

Chapter 15

Preparing the Construction Site

Earlier in the book an article was referenced that stated that most people do not know what they are doing in a gym. If that described you, things are about to change because a series of foundational exercises will be clearly demonstrated for you. In addition, a video is available through the *www.fitfooddude.com* website that thoroughly covers everything for those of you who are visual and auditory learners. Plus, in the back of the book, other credible books and websites are listed to help those seeking to add variety to their workout programs. For now, though, the exercises in this book can serve most of you quite well for the first year, if not for a lifetime. Follow them and perform them consistently, correctly and enthusiastically and you will soon be in the top 5% of fitness levels for your age.

An attempt has been made to be a little different than other books on strength training. Virtually every strength-training book you can find will cover and demonstrate a myriad of strength training exercises. That is a good thing for those who already have some strength training experience. In this book, though, the goal is for you to learn *at least one* of the standard exercises for each major muscle group of the body. Exercises you may have never seen before are included. They are included because they are great for getting results, allow you to progress from easier to more difficult, and they keep things interesting by using a variety of movements to stimulate muscle groups.

Several of the movements are highly effective in increasing functionality. Functionality basically means how our bodies operate in every day activities, such as getting out of a chair, lifting things overhead from shelves, working in the yard, climbing stairs, etc. The exercises that show alternating movements of arms or legs are especially effective to this end. By their nature, alternating movements require greater stabilization of the body and rotation of the spinal column. As such, they help to increase our ability to do everything more safely and aggressively. As we build our bodies in this fashion, we can confidently stay active throughout our lives and enjoy more of the fruits of a healthiness lifestyle.

One way to know if something is working and that you are making progress is to keep score. Before you start, it is important to clearly write down your goals. A goal setting form has been included that has proven effective for many people. But it is important to use several tools to help you keep score, so that you can see how your game is progressing. Do not overlook this step. Can you imagine watching a sporting event where no score was kept? It would get boring rather quickly wouldn't it? By establishing our fitness baseline and then working to improving it, we can take advantage of this intrinsic drive and keep ourselves motivated and interested in how we are doing. You can either hire a trainer to help you with this (see references) or simply review and do the following:

Before you start the program:

1) **Visit your doctor.** Get their permission to exercise first! I would recommend that you take this book to your doctor and show them the exercises in this book. Feel free to have them contact me at

fitfooddude@aol.com if they have any questions or comments. Then, get a blood test, along with blood pressure, body weight, resting heart rate, and bodyweight measurements. Keep records of these stored away for now. Approximately three months after starting, revisit your doctor to note improvements!

2) **Measurements**. Invest in a good tape measure for your body. They are inexpensive, but valuable, and better than any scale will ever be. I have referenced a company in the back to help with this (www.accufitness.com), or they can be purchased through my website. The measurement information on page 204 is similar to the information I used thirty years ago when I first began training. It will serve to motivate and encourage you as you progress. Please **DO NOT** use it to beat yourself up if you don't see major progress right away. Keep working at it, and you will soon see and feel the rewards.

3) **Body fat measurement**. (Optional). Body fat skin-fold measurements can be done by a trainer, or you can do it yourself. Body fat measurement can be made a complex task, or simple. I think most of us prefer simple. Just purchase body fat calipers ($16.-$20.) and then learn how to take a single, uncomplicated measurement, above your right hipbone. The calipers I recommend come with a small instruction book, and you purchase them at www.accufitness.com or at www.fitfooddude.com. There are scales that measure both bodyweight and body fat percentage. They can be rather expensive and are generally less accurate than calipers. However, they are better than nothing and can indicate whether your body fat is increasing or decreasing.

4) **Take a picture**. (Optional). Yes, this is not primarily about appearance, but our health is often reflected on the outside as well. This is only for you to look back on a year or two from now. Many people feel uncomfortable getting their pictures taken, especially in just a pair of shorts (men) or a swimsuit. Yet, several trainees who failed to take a picture initially, expressed regret a

year or so later that they had not done this. If you do take pictures, take one from the front, back and side views. Then, put them away in a safe place, or for the bolder, on the front of your refrigerator!

As you progress through your workouts and improving your eating habits, you will keep records as well. Forms for doing so are included in later sections of this book. It is especially important to track your workouts, as each progression you make in weight used, repetitions, distance and time can be correlated to an improvement in your overall health.

5) Familiarize yourself with the basic anatomy of muscles
The pictures below outline the very basic major muscle groups on the human body, both for women and men. Take a little time to become familiar with them. There are over 600 muscles on the body, and each is important. But for our intents and purposes, the ones outlined will suffice. In truth, we will be focusing for the most part on entire body segments, such as muscles that push and pull the upper body, and those that push and pull the lower body. This is perhaps oversimplifying it a bit, but is all we truly need to know to be spectacularly successful.

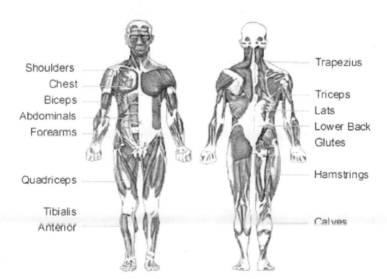

Shoulders
Chest
Biceps
Abdominals
Forearms

Quadriceps

Tibialis
Anterior

Trapezius

Triceps
Lats
Lower Back
Glutes

Hamstrings

Calves

6) Get the basic equipment. Although it is possible to start without equipment, it is not the best way to go. The workouts outlined are all designed to be able to be done at your home. They can be done at the gym as well, of course, but the intent is for anyone to be able to perform them without joining a gym, or buying highly expensive equipment. For those of you who want to join a gym or buy one of the more expensive home gyms, these workouts can be adapted to your situation as well.

One of the objections often heard at conferences is, "you mean I have to spend money to buy equipment? Can't I just use soup cans or milk cartons?" My response is this. We are talking about your body, your health and your life. Then I give the, "spend a little money on yourself" lecture. People spend all kinds of money on couches and other household furniture. What has your couch ever really done for you? What did you pay for it? Unless you bought it at a yard sale, it likely cost you more than $200.

Some books say to use soup cans, etc in place of real weights. These authors are recommending less than the best. One of the problems with these types of objects is that it is difficult to measure progression. "Hey Bob; guess what, I went from lifting Campbell's chicken noodle 8 oz to extra thick and chunky 12 oz". I don't think so. Using such items to me seems like a mediocre commitment. You can't walk on water unless you get out of the boat. Invest in your health. Buy some decent equipment. You can get started with weight training rather inexpensively. Most women can pick up enough weights to keep them challenged for under $50 at your local Wal-Mart. Speaking of yard sales, spend a week or two reading the classifieds. I have found some great deals on weights in the paper. Just don't buy any fitness fantasy gizmos instead!

For those of you **looking for the best**, the Powerblock Company (*www.powerblock.com*) carries excellent dumbbell sets that can meet anyone's strength levels. There are different size sets to meet all strength levels, and most of their sets are interchangeable so that you can add-on as your strength increases. Yes, they are more costly. Think about it though. If the transmission on your car went out today, it would most likely cost you at least $1000 to get it fixed. And, though it might be tough, you would somehow find the money to complete the repair. Why? Because you need your car!! You need your body even more. Buy good equipment and follow the programs in this book. Chances of your bodies "transmission" going out will be greatly reduced.

It is highly recommended buying an adjustable weight bench as well. You can make good progress without one, but eventually it is something you will want to pick up. Again, most local sporting goods stores run sales on these, or the newspaper can be a good source. The bench does not have to be gym quality, just sturdy enough to support your bodyweight safely. You could get by with a flat bench, but an adjustable bench that inclines and goes upright is best. I recently saw a bench at Wal-Mart that would be great for most of us. It was a "powerhouse model sb210-multi-function bench." The price was about $40.00. No, I do not own any Wal-Mart stock. One other small piece of equipment you will need is a timer. Stop watches are fine of course, but I like to use a standard kitchen timer with an alarm of when my time is up!

More Workout Details . . .

A) **Warm-ups:** Before starting to exercise, warming up a little is always a good idea. Doing so is like sending a message to the body that some effort above and beyond the normal is coming. The point of warming up is to get blood flowing to the muscle groups to be worked. The blood is what "warms" the muscle up, as well as sends oxygen to the muscles to be worked. The best way to warm up is to do so with the same exercise that will be used in the workout, but at a slower pace. For example, my first strength training exercise is usually incline dumbbell presses. I perform my first set with a relatively light weight, and focus on lifting and lowering the weight slowly, through the complete range, while breathing deeply. This is enough for me and my body, and seems to be enough for most people I know. If you require more, perform 10-15 jumping jacks or pushups and you should be good to go.

B) **Stretching**: Years ago the thought was that stretching before exercise was beneficial. Reality is though that stretching cold muscles does not prevent either soreness or injury. Rather, stretching before exercising or working out may actually increase chances of injury in that it temporarily weakens the muscles. I personally prefer full range body weight exercises to improve flexibility, but do recommend a few stretches to be performed **after** your workout.

C) **Rest periods**: In order to get the best results form strength training, keep your rest periods between exercises brief. One minute is ideal, and I recommend that you utilize a stop-watch or kitchen timer to keep yourself honest and on track. If you find yourself particularly winded after an exercise, you may rest up to two minutes, but any longer than that is not suggested. Remember we discussed the fact that strength training is great for the health of your heart, just as aerobic exercise is. One of the keys to realizing strength trainings benefits is to keep the rest periods brief. For extra intensity, you can reduce rest between sets to thirty seconds. But again, one minute is ideal for most.

D) **Amount of weight**: One of the most frequent questions received is, "how much weight should I use?" This is a tough question to answer for any one individual. Rather, the amount of weight used will vary from person to person. The rule of thumb is this. For all upper body exercises, find a weight that you can lift 10 times (repetitions) using proper technique. This means a weight that requires no excessive straining or jerking, one that you can smoothly raise in 4 seconds and lower in 4 seconds, but starts becoming more and more difficult as you progress towards 10. The 9th and 10th lifts, movements or repetitions should become difficult to complete. Many men attempt to use too much weight before they know how to properly perform the exercise. Most women, on the other hand, consistently use too little of a weight. Be sure to learn the proper methods first, and the strength is sure to follow if the workouts are followed consistently and correctly.

With the proper amount of weight, you will be able to lift it 10 times, but if you were to attempt to lift it 11 times, it would be doubtful that you could. With the proper amount of weight, it should feel that at 10 reps, you could no longer continue, and need to take a one-minute rest. As your strength improves to the point that lifting the weight 12-15 times is possible, it is time to increase the weights by 1.25-2.5 pounds. Above I mentioned that many men attempt to lift too much weight too soon. The opposite, as I said is true of many women. One of the biggest frustrations of trainers in working with many women is that they are too fearful of lifting heavier weights, thus missing out on achieving their true health and fitness potential. This, most likely, is due to the old myths of getting muscles like a man, etc.

Hopefully, that has been put to rest at this point. Still, I talk with so many women who say they are strength training, yet the heaviest weights they are lifting is a 3-5 pound dumbbell. Then, they lift their 20-25 pound child 5-10 times a day, no problem! If you can lift a dumbbell more than 10 times, think about increasing the weight. Staying with a 3-5 pound dumbbell when it is possible for you to lift 15-25 pounds or more is not really doing much for you at all.

E) **Technique:** Fitness infomercial guru Tony Little wrote a book called, "Technique", and on his old shows he could be heard yelling, "technique, technique" at his clients much of the time. On this point, I agree with Tony Little, although whether yelling it in a person's ear continuously works I'm not sure. But, the point is well taken. If you are not performing the exercise correctly, you are not getting all the benefit you can. And, I believe that 80% of those working out in most gyms are not using correct technique, based upon my observations. Learning the correct technique, however, takes time and practice. Like any new physical endeavor, at the start it may feel awkward. Like a Golf swing, at first it feels a little hesitant and jerky, but over time becomes more natural and smooth. Study this book, try the exercises, refer back to the pictures, and keep at it. You may want to hire a trainer for a workout or two to help you learn the methods, or purchase our video and follow along as we demonstrate the exercises for you. But do not give up. These exercises are a gold mine, a super lotto for your body, if you will just be tenacious and stay with it.

F) **Intensity**: This is a difficult subject to address, but it feels necessary to briefly review it. Intensity is related to how hard one works, the amount of physical and mental effort brought to a task at hand. The amount of weight we use determines in part how hard we will work, but other factors such as the speed of movements we employ, number of repetitions and sets, all affect our physical efforts. And, using the proper amounts of all of these variables is important to our success. I would like to focus, however, on our mental effort. Time will be spent later on in the book on mental attitude, but before we start the workouts it is important to mention that what we get out of these workouts, like all in life, depends upon what we put in. As you go through the workouts, focus in on the muscles, and utilize your best mental determination to push yourself at the highest level of safety. This is, of course, after you are confident that you know how to correctly perform the exercise and have done so a few times with a light weight. If you need a trainer at first to help you reach that level, so be it. But, to get our best for ourselves, the advice of my high school football coach applies here. He continuously told us, "Don't be a wheelbarrow". In other words, don't rely on others to pick you up and carry you. Do it yourself, and for yourself at first. Then, later on, you can help others to do the same!

G) **Eating:** When, how much, and what you eat before exercising depends on when you will workout. Most experts tell you to eat a small carbohydrate meal before you workout, preferably 2 hours or so before working out. Other experts say to have a small protein meal one to 1.5 hours before working out, followed by a carbohydrate meal right after your workout to replace glycogen that was used up. And if you workout first thing in the morning, you may want to not eat anything before your workout, but within 30 minutes of completing your workout. In truth, I have used all three methods, and have found all three to be successful. My personal favorite, however, is to eat a small protein meal one to 1.5 hours before exercising. And for me, it is virtually always the same.

I mix two scoops of mocha flavored whey protein, a tablespoon of heavy whipping cream and coffee and drink it about one hour in advance of my workout. Then, immediately after my workout, I have a meal of straight carbohydrates to replace the glycogen used up during exercise. Sometimes my pre-workout meal might be a few tablespoons of natural peanut butter, or an orange. Both of those are easy for me to digest, and don't affect my ability to workout hard. On those days that I workout immediately upon waking up, I will simply have a cup of black coffee, and eat immediately after my workout. If possible though, it is optimum to eat before you workout (1.5-2 hours is best), keep it light and devoid of any excess heavy fats.

H) **Breathing:** It is important that you breathe properly when exercising. Rule of thumb is to *exhale* when raising or pulling against resistance and inhale as you go back to the starting position.

I) **Repetition**: the number of times you lift and lower weight in one set of an exercise. For example, if you lift and lower a weight 10 times before setting the weight down, you have completed 10 "reps" in one set.

J) **Set**: a group of repetitions (raising/pulling and lowering resistance) of an exercise after which you take a brief rest (30 seconds to one minute is recommended).

K) **Training to failure:** This is actually the "secret" to success, and the primary difference between those who get great results and those who do not. When you train to failure, you raise and lower the weight until you are sure you cannot do another repetition, also known as "momentary muscular failure". For example, lets say that I am doing arm curls with a 25 lb dumbbell. My goal is to lift it 10 times. By the time I reach my 7th rep, however, my arms start feeling fatigued. I decide to keep going though, knowing that this is when the most benefit takes place. I continue to maintain proper exercise form, breathe deeply and correctly, and maintain a nice slow, steady pace. Through focus and determination I manage to reach 10 reps and, though it's really hard, I am still able to continue moving the weight. So I keep going, even though little beads of sweat are forming on my forehead! Finally, at 12 reps, I cannot move the weight one inch further. I now lower the weight slowly, back to the beginning position.

Caution

While Training to failure is best, it is not always for everyone, all of the time. If you are new to training, are in injury rehabilitation, or have a chronic disease that is not conducive to excessive strain at this time, start by simply doing the movements at a medium level of effort. Training to failure is the way to maximal results, and most people do not know this. But it is better to be training some, than not at all. So, start with reasonable efforts, and when you feel ready, you can begin to push yourself a little harder.

Training to failure is tougher than what most of us are used to. Others and I do it that way, because we know it produces. Still, there are days where I do not train to failure. Perhaps the baby was up late, and I'm short on sleep, etc. That being the case, I take it a little easy in my workout, knowing that I can push myself harder next workout.

L) **Tempo**: This is also a big key to avoiding injury and getting the best results. If you adhere to the tempo of 4 seconds to raise and 4 seconds to lower, maintain strict form and do not cheat (arching of back, bouncing or yanking of weights, excessive grimacing and teeth clenching, yelling, etc), you should be able to continue with this exercise method for the rest of your life. Slow and steady wins the race.

M) **Get a reliable workout partner**: Partners have only a 6% dropout rate. Those who go it alone?? 43%!

N) **Music/environment**: Play your favorite upbeat music that inspires you! If you train at home, make your exercise area invigorating.

O) **Enthusiasm**: Build enthusiasm, the world needs more of it regarding a fitness lifestyle (and everything else). Remember the "Little Engine That Could".

P) **Time**: This is your time. Guard it tenaciously. Take care of yourself so that you can be prepared to take care of others as well. If you do not have time for this in your life, your life may be too busy, and you may want to rethink your priorities and what less productive activities can be done away with or reduced.

Q) **Goals**: Set your goals in writing. Join the top 2%!! Remember the "reticular activating system" and that FORM FOLLOWS FUNCTION. Goal setting forms are found on pages 295-296 and 299.

R) **Keep Records**: Keep score. Feedback is the breakfast of champions. A sample workout scorecard is found on page 201.

S) **Time of day:** Many people want to know the best time of day to train. The best time to train for most people is early in the morning, for three primary reasons. First, doing so jump-starts your metabolism for the day. Second, it also boosts your mood through the release of endorphins into your bloodstream. Remember the power of endorphins. They are the strongest anti-depressant and pain-killer known. And the third reason is that if you train early, the chances of something "coming up" to interfere with your training time are reduced. Still, any time of day that works for you will work. I have heard of people who train in the evening, but when I have done so, it has affected my sleep adversely, likely due to an elevated metabolism.

T) **Training Days:** It is recommended you strength train three days per week. This is especially true if it is the only exercise you are doing. Several studies have shown that you can get good results from only two strength training sessions per week, and if you are using other exercise forms on non-strength training days, that would be o.k. If you train twice per week, split it up with a two-day break in between. For example, Monday and Thursday. It would be *best* to strength train 3 days though. Most people who do so train Mon-Wed-Fri or Sat-Tues-Thur. Do not strength train two days in a row. Weight lifting impacts your body at a deeper level than other forms of exercise, and your body needs time to reconstruct it self.

Personally, I lift weights and do aerobic exercise on the same day, three days per week (Mon-Wed-Fri). Then, I do a few minutes of body weight exercises on alternate days (Sat-Tues-Thurs), and take Sundays off. I have spent many years studying and trying what works best. I believe I have found it. Follow it as you see *FIT!*

U) **Difficulty of exercises:** Most exercise books will categorize the exercises as beginner, advanced, etc. That has not been done in this book. The reason being is that all of the exercises can benefit anyone, even the "advanced" trainer. I consider myself advanced, and made the mistake for several years of not doing some exercises that I considered to be for "beginners". I have since learned that by focusing effort, any exercise can be made challenging and beneficial. Still, some of the exercises are a little tougher, and in those cases a note has been made of that in the instructions. If in doubt on your ability to perform an exercise, spend some time practicing the movement with no or very little resistance. If it is beyond your ability for now, so be it. Find another movement you can do that works the same muscles, and master it. When the time is right, come back to the more challenging one and try again.

V) **Machines or free weights?** This is one of the great debates in the world of strength training and fitness. Some experts feel that all beginners (especially seniors and those recovering from injury) should start on machines. That is not a bad idea, but there are a few "issues" with it. First, many people do not have access to a gym or equipment. All of the exercises demonstrated in this book can be done with either dumbbells or no weight at all. Thus, anyone can do these in his or her own home. The second issue with machines is that they do not provide as much functional or stability training as free weights (barbells and dumbbells). This is especially true compared to dumbbells. Functional and stability training basically means that the exercise more closely mimics movements we perform in real life and requires the use of "stabilizer" muscles. Stabilizer muscles are those that assist the larger muscles and hold everything together. For example, when doing a set of one-armed straddle rows (page 160), not only is the target muscle of the upper back involved. Rather, the hamstrings, lower back, abs, etc all help to hold the body in balance as the exercise is performed. Also, that particular exercise helps the body for any real life activity that requires bending and lifting.

That cannot be said of machines. Machines do have advantages however. First, they can be quite safe. Most anyone can use them with a little guidance. But I have actually seen this benefit backfire. Some gym trainers assume that people don't need much instruction on machines, and forego giving enough instruction to novice trainees, Thus, we see people yanking and overexerting on machines that are supposed to be safer. Another problem I have seen with machines is that people get so used to them; they never take the next step to learn how to train with free weights, and specifically, dumbbells.

For my money, if I could have only one piece of exercise equipment, it would be dumbbells. They offer you the most benefit and variety, and can accomplish *any* fitness goal. When I was learning to drive, my father taught me on a four-wheel drive stick shift international scout, with no power steering (or power anything for that matter). He said, "If you can learn to drive this, you will be able to drive anything." Learn to do the exercises in this book, with or without the dumbbells, and you will be able to transfer that knowledge to exercise effectively anywhere, anytime, and on any equipment.

W) **Cardio/Aerobic Exercise:** Our focus for now is on learning and doing these strength-training exercises. The first goal is to make them a habitual part of your lifestyle. As said before, there were times in my life, when all I did was strength train, and was in very good condition. For those who want to take it to the next level, though, you will want to add some cardio work eventually. The one point I want to make at this time is that cardio is always done AFTER strength training. We will discuss cardio in more detail in the upcoming workout chapter.

Section V

Help Your Body Win . . .
The Workout

Chapter 16

The Workout . . . Where the Rubber

Meets the Road.

*No discipline seems pleasant at the time, but painful. Later
on, however, it produces a harvest of righteousness and peace
for those who have been **trained** by it. Therefore, strengthen
your feeble arms and weak knees.*

Hebrews 12:11-12

Always check with your Doctor before starting any exercise program.

Let's Get To It!

You will strength train 3 days per week, every other day, for
approximately 25-30 minutes per session, followed by 10-15
minutes of cardio exercise (45 minutes total). Usually this means
Mon-Wed-Fri or Tues-Thurs-Sat. Your program will consist of 10
exercises. No more, no less. Your program will always be built on
a foundation of 3 exercises. One upper body pushing movement,
one upper body pulling movement, and one lower body movement.
This allows for *thoroughly* working all of the major muscle groups

of the body, which is our goal. Each of these foundational exercises will be done twice per workout, for 10-15 repetitions, unless specified otherwise.

For example, I recommend the incline dumbbell press as one of the best upper body push exercises. You would start with a weight or resistance for this exercise that you could complete for 10-12 repetitions. You would do this once, and let's say you complete 12 repetitions on the first try. Then, after a 60 second rest period, you complete a second "set". On this second set you are only able to do 9 repetitions. For now, you should stay with this weight. We will stay with this weight until you are able to complete 15 reps on the first set and at least ten on the second set. When you have reached these numbers (using proper form and safety), it is time to increase your resistance by 1-5 lbs. This same progression will apply to all exercises listed, unless the exercise is a bodyweight only exercise. In that case, one could either keep adding repetitions or slow down the speed of the movement, which makes it more challenging.

The foundational, primary exercises we will use are broken down according to the body **sections** described above. They are upper body *push muscles,* which consist of the chest, front shoulder and triceps. Next is upper body *pull*, which consists of the broader upper back muscles known as the lats, the trapezius, which is the trapezoid shaped muscle running from the base of the neck to the shoulders and mid-back, the rear shoulders, biceps, and forearms. And third, are the lower body muscles, which include the gluteus or butt, the front and back of the thighs (quadriceps and hamstrings), the lower leg or calves, and the lower back.

After the foundational exercises are listed, we then move to the assistive exercises, which are muscles and movements that "assist" the larger muscle groups. These exercises focus on the triceps, biceps, shoulder joint, hip joint and knee joint. I generally recommend these exercises be performed only once, in order to keep our workout schedule at 10 exercises. A person can pick and choose from these "assistive" exercises, depending upon their individual goals and needs. We have demonstrated all of the exercise with photos and have provided a "scorecard" for you to use to insure you are following the program and keeping track of your progress.

On the scorecard included, the first six exercise types suggested are marked for you. The other four slots are left blank. Look at the assistive exercises and select a few to include in your workouts that seem as if they would help you the most. For instance, if your knees are weak, you may want to do the leg extensions demonstrated on page184. Or if you'd like to strengthen and tighten the back of your upper arms, include one of the triceps exercises. Are you ready? Good, let's get started!

Exercise Models

The "models' in these photos include myself, my 9 year old daughter, my 16 year old son and my mother in law. My daughter uses light weights to strengthen her body, help her develop coordination and enhance her dancing ability. My son works out to prepare for his high school football team and because he wants to feel and look his best. You know my story. My mother-in-law is in the process of fighting for her fitness future after a 2 year battle with cancer.

UPPER BODY *PUSH* EXERCISES
(Pick one from this category.)

Utilizes the pushing muscle groups of the upper body, the chest (pectorals), back of the upper arms (triceps), and the front/middle shoulder muscles (deltoids). I recommend changing the exercises every four weeks or so. This is done for two reasons, first, to keep thing interesting mentally and second, to challenge the muscles from different angles. Having said that, if there is a movement I really like (incline chest press with dumbbells), I will stay with it for several months before mixing things up.

Incline Chest Press:

Function: Upper body push
Muscles: Upper chest, front shoulders, triceps
Repetitions: 10-15

* This is perhaps my personal favorite upper body **push** exercise. It provides a good stretch of the shoulders and rib cage.

1) Set your bench as close as possible to midway between flat and straight up.

2) Start by picking up a dumbbell in each hand and then sit down on the incline bench.

3) Lift the dumbbells, one at a time, to shoulder level, with your palms facing forward, lean back into the bench and steady yourself.

4) Slowly push the weights (4 sec) up, while exhaling, at the top, pause slightly, slowly (4 sec) lower weights while inhaling. Pause briefly (no more than one second) and continue.

5) When you can lift the weight properly between 11-15 times, add about 2.5 pounds the next time you workout.

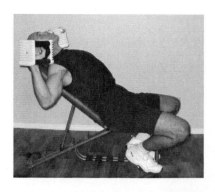
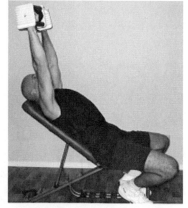

Bench Press Flat

Function: Upper body push
Muscles: Chest, Front Shoulders, Triceps (Back of upper arms)
Repetitions:10-12

A) Lying flat on a bench or the floor, begin this exercise with two dumbbells held above shoulders, arms extended and elbows slightly flexed.
B) Slowly lower the dumbbells, with your elbows turned outward, until your upper arms are parallel to the floor.
C) Avoid dropping your elbows too far below the bench.
D) Pause in the lower position for a moment, and then slowly raise the dumbbells back to the starting position.

* For variation, try alternating arms.

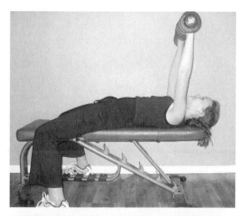

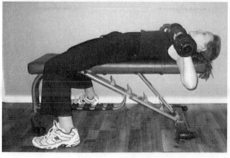

Shoulder press

Function: Upper body push
Muscles: Shoulders, trapezius, triceps
Repetitions: 12-18

* This exercise can be done seated or standing. If you stand, maintain an erect posture with knees slightly bent, feet about shoulder width apart. For variation and increased strengthening of the spine, alternate arms when lifting.

1) Sit with good posture on a bench or solid chair (preferably against a backrest)
2) Lift both dumbbells upward to the starting position, so they are on either side of your head with your palms facing inward.
3) Slowly (4 seconds) begin to push both (or alternate) dumbbells upward with your elbows turned outward.
4) Do not lock your elbows or arch your back in the upper position. Keep your head level to the ground.
5) Pause briefly in the upper position, then slowly lower back to the starting position.

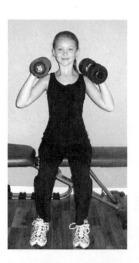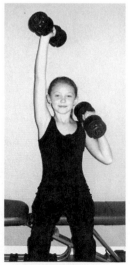

Pushups

Function: Upper body push
Muscles: Chest, front of shoulders, triceps, stabilizer muscles (lower back, abs)
Repetitions: 4-25

1) Push body away from floor, keeping legs, back and head in a straight line.
2) Pause slightly at the top, and slowly lower until your chest brushes the floor.
3) Be sure to breathe properly, exhaling as you push, inhale as you lower.
4) If you are unable to do these correctly, start by lowering yourself only from the finish position (On toes and hands with body stiff). Once you reach the floor, get back to the top and lower yourself again. Stay with it for at least 4 reps. This is a great exercise that is often overlooked because it has been around so long. Learn to love these, and you will always be able to workout, no matter where you are!!

* In this photo, I am using a band for added resistance.

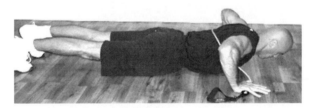

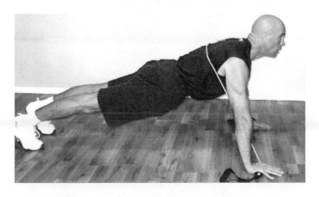

Standing Push-offs

Function: Upper Body Push
Muscles: Chest, front of shoulders, triceps, lower back, abdominal muscles (stabilization)
Repetitions: 10-25

1) Stand with feet 16 inches apart about 3 feet away from desk, countertop or wall.
2) Place hands about shoulder width apart at chest level or a bit lower on desk, etc.
3) Arms are extended & straight, inhale and lower forward, bending arms at elbow until chest almost touches. You may stand on your toes for better range of motion.
4) Keep legs, knees, and torso in straight alignment, return to start while exhaling.

   o   I once thought this was too wimpy. I found though, that by going slower & focusing on the chest muscles, it gets the job done. If it's too easy, shoot to do 50! This is a great one for hotel workouts. By moving hands closer together, really hits the triceps.

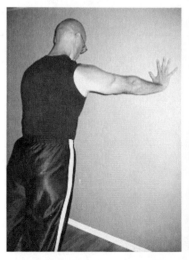 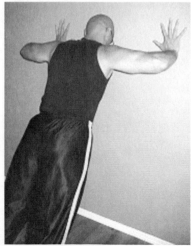

Chair Pushups

Function: Upper body push
Muscles: Chest, front shoulders, upper back, triceps
Repetitions: 1-50

1) Get two sturdy, non-slip chairs
2) Place them about shoulder width apart
3) Place hands securely on inside edge of chairs, legs straight behind, back straight, head up.
4) Keep body rigid; lower yourself *slowly* as far as you can go.
5) Pause at the bottom, and then press to starting position. Inhale down, exhale up.

*This is my second favorite chest exercise. It really hits the muscles but also provides a great stretch for the entire upper body and gets blood flow going deep into the muscle fibers. Work into it slowly though, as it requires a higher degree of strength.

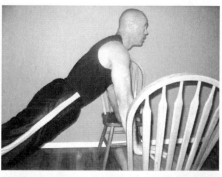

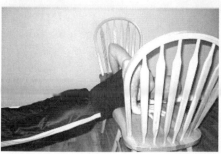

UPPER BODY *PULL* EXERCISES
(Pick one from this category.)

The muscles primarily required for these exercises include the lats (broad upper back muscles), rear shoulders, trapezius (runs from mid-back to shoulder joints to base of neck). Biceps, forearms and lower back also are involved. These muscles assist in everyday living, a high metabolism and good posture.

One arm rows, straddle:

Function: Upper body pull
Muscles: Lats (upper back), back of shoulders, trapezius, biceps, forearm, hand grip, glutes, lower back.
Repetitions: 10-15

1) Bend knees, keep back flat, place left elbow on left knee.
2) Hold dumbbell, palm in at arms length, about six inches from floor.
3) Pull dumbbell straight up to side of lower torso, keeping arm close to side.
4) Return to starting position using same path.
5) Exhale as you raise the weight, inhale as you lower. Reverse positions and repeat movement on the left side

* This movement hits the lower back and glute (butt) also, and will make starting your lawn mower or chain saw much easier.

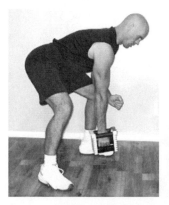 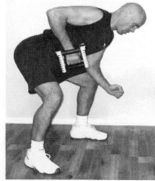

One Arm Row, supported

Function: Upper Body Pull
Muscles: Lats, Shoulders, Trapezius, Lower Back, Biceps
Repetitions: 10-15

* This is a good one for those who currently have lower back weakness & cannot perform the straddle row comfortably

1) Grip a dumbbell in your right hand.
2) Place your left knee and left hand on the bench.
3) Keep your right knee slightly bent and your back flat throughout the exercise.
4) Draw the dumbbell upward toward the lower ribs, keeping elbow close to body.
5) Pause in the upper position for a moment, and then slowly lower (4 seconds) the dumbbell back down until your arm is fully extended.
6) Perform a set on the right side, and then switch to your left side.

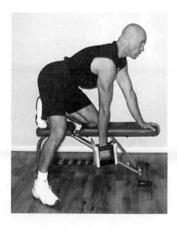
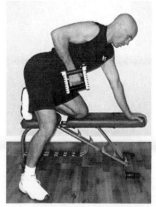

Upright Row

Function: Upper body pull
Muscles: Shoulders, trapezius, biceps, forearms
Repetitions: 12-18

1) Stand with feet comfortably apart, knees slightly bent.
2) Hold both dumbbells in front of body, palms facing you.
3) Begin lifting one weight upward, keeping it parallel to the ground.
4) Continue lifting to mid chest line, pause for a moment, and then slowly lower back to the starting position. Do not lift the weights higher than mid-chest. Doing so places strain on shoulder joints. Keep weights close to the body and move them smoothly and slowly with no jerking.
5) Repeat with opposite arm and alternate until done.

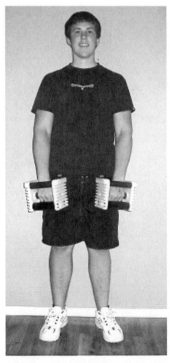 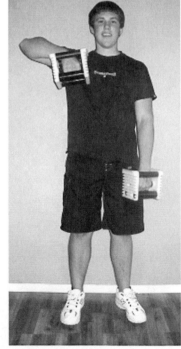

LOWER BODY
(Pick one from this category.)

These exercises affect all of the muscles, joints, tendons and ligaments of the lower body. This includes the glutes (butt), front and rear thighs, lower leg, and lower back. The lower body is the foundation of our "house" and affects our health and fitness in a major way. Work hard on all of the exercises, but give these ones a little extra "umph".

Stationary lunge

Function: Improves lower body strength and function
Muscle areas: Glutes (butt), Quadriceps (front upper thigh), Hamstrings (back of upper thigh), Lower back, Calves, Tibialis Anterior (front of lower leg).
Repetitions: 10-20 (Start exercise with no weight until 20 are easy)

*Only lower yourself as far as you can comfortably go until your strength improves.

1) Stand to the back and side of a bench or chair with feet shoulder width apart. Hold on lightly to back of bench (or any stable object) with free hand.

2) Take a medium step forward with right leg. Your feet will be about 3-4 feet apart. Keep your right knee over your right foot, but not past your toes. Your left knee will bend slightly, and your left heel will come up slightly off the floor.

3) Now, *slowly* lower yourself, dropping your hips until your back knee nearly touches the floor (or, as far as you can go for now. Do not concern yourself too much with how far you can go. As your strength grows, you will be able to go further). Keep your head up, chest out, upper body erect.

4) Pause for one second, and then push your self back into the starting position. Focus on pushing through the heels while keeping toes

on the ground. Complete the recommended reps with one leg,
and then switch to the other leg.

* This is one of my favorite lower body exercises, although it will
be a challenge for many. Still, if everyone in America did this
throughout their lives, there would be far fewer unhealthy and/or
obese people and far fewer people in nursing homes. This exercise
can help us stay lean, active for a lifetime! Learn it, live it, love it.

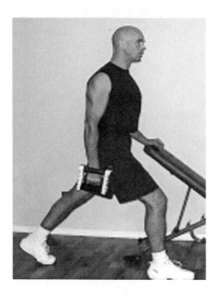

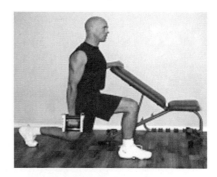

Deep knee bends

Function: Lower body strength and function
Muscles improved: Glutes, thighs, calves, lower back and abs
Repetitions: 10-100

1) Stand erect with arms held straight out in front for balance
2) Keeping eyes straight ahead, bend at the knees and lower yourself all the way to the floor.
3) As you lower yourself, rise up on your toes.
4) Pause for a brief second and return to the starting position.

At first, some of you may find this exercise tough, but stay with it. It *may* never get easy, but it will get easier. These are great not only for strength, but *flexibility* and stamina in the legs as well. In addition, as you will see, this exercise is an excellent cardiovascular exercise. It will likely get you huffing and puffing as well as anything you can imagine, and that is good! It can be done anywhere and anytime as well. I sometimes do these while barbecuing in the backyard. If you have knee problems, lower yourself slowly to see how it feels. Most everyone can eventually do this. It is an *awesome* exercise, and perhaps the number one exercise you can do for your lower body strength, endurance and health. Some fitness experts have warned about lowering your self this far, because of the strain on the knees. The problem is not that this is dangerous though; the problem is that our knees and legs have become weak and inflexible through inactivity.

If you watch a toddler, they spend a lot of time crouched on their knees. Likewise, I have seen farm workers in my hometown stay in this position for long periods of time as they harvest strawberries. Our legs were meant to function in this way. We have simply stopped using them for this function! I am 45 years old and have abused my legs as much or more than most, yet I can still crank out 50 of these, no problem. I am confident you will soon be joining me. I learned this exercise from a book back in the early 70's, and have not found any other machine, etc, that can beat it. If your knees crack and pop, that is not usually a need for concern but rather a sign that your tendons and ligaments need strengthening and more blood flow to that area. If you experience sharp pain *in your joints*, however, do the flat-footed or chair squats for now. Attempt to do 20 of these. When 20 becomes doable, aim for 50, 75, 100. Have fun.

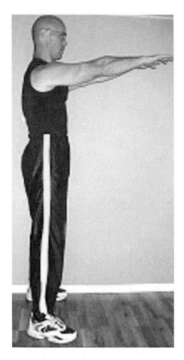
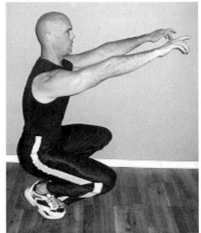

FREEHAND FLATFOOTED SQUATS
(no weights used)

Function: Improves the lower body
Muscles: Glutes, thighs, lower leg, lower back. Abs
Repetitions: 15-20

1) Stand with arms extended in front of you or crossed over the chest
2) Head up, back straight, feet 16 inches apart.
3) Lower yourself slowly while inhaling, until thighs are parallel to the floor.
4) Head stays up, back straight, knees slightly out, hold briefly
5) Return to starting position

- o Feet stay flat on the floor in this exercise. Inhale and exhale deeply for the full benefit!
- o When you can easily do 20 of these, move on to the deep knee bends or dumbbell squats.

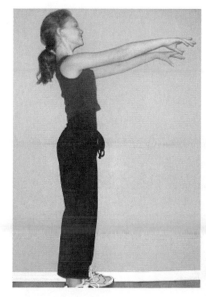
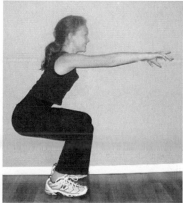

Dumbbell squats

Function: Improves function and appearance of lower body
Muscles: Glutes, Thighs (quadriceps and hamstrings), lower back and legs, abs
Repetitions: 10-20

1) Grip a dumbbell in each hand and hold at or rest on the shoulder.
2) Stand with feet shoulder width apart, knees slightly bent, and toes pointed slightly out.
3) Slowly lower your hips until your upper thighs are almost parallel to the floor.
4) Pause at the bottom and slowly return to the standing position, straightening your legs and hips at the same time.
5) Keep your back flat or with a slight arch, throughout the exercise.
6) Keep your feet firmly on the floor and squat only as low as you can with proper technique. Use very little weight the first time you perform this exercise.

   o   If you have difficulty balancing, use a 2 in board or similar object under your heels.

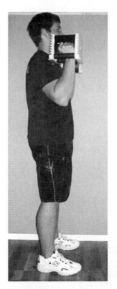 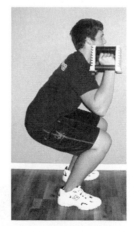

Squats to a bench or chair

Function: Improves lower body function and appearance
Muscles: Glutes, thighs, lower back and legs, abs
Repetitions: 10-20

1) Stand 16" in front of bench, arms crossed over chest
2) Head up, back straight, feet 16" apart
3) Squat until buttocks touches bench, inhaling as you lower
4) Keep tension on thighs; do not rest on bench
5) Head stays up, back straight, knees slightly out
6) Return to starting position, exhaling as you come up

    o   If you find this too unstable, you may want to place
        your bench/chair near a door. Then with the door open,
        hold on to the door handle from both sides for support
        as you raise and lower yourself. This is a very safe way
        for anyone to get started doing squats.

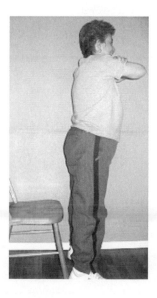
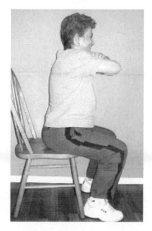

Balance Lunge

Function: Improves Lower body function, flexibility, balance and appearance.

Muscles: Special emphasis on the hamstrings, thighs, glutes

Repetitions: 8-12

o   This is a tough one. Do not attempt this until you can comfortably perform 20 full range stationary lunges with dumbbells. Still, it will hit your muscles and challenge them at a higher level.

1) Place right foot on a bench or chair. Step forward with left foot about 3 feet, lightly holding onto support with your right hand.
2) Be sure to keep left knee directly above left ankle. Do not let left knee extend in front of your toes.
3) Keeping upper body straight, eyes ahead, chest out. Slowly drop hips straight down, while bending at left knee. Take it slow, as this is tough. The farthest you will want to go is when your left thigh is parallel to the floor. Pause for a moment, ask yourself why you are doing this, and then return to the starting position.
4) Complete the reps with this leg, and then switch to the other leg.

☺   And, the reason you are doing this exercise, is because it is so good for your fitness future!

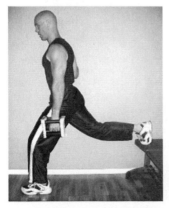 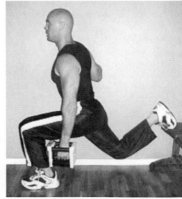

ASSISTIVE EXERCISES
(Pick up to four from this group.)

Muscle Specific

These exercises will round out the ten needed for your program. The dilemma here is that everyone is different and has different needs. So many of the people I meet have special challenges with different parts of their body. Issues such as bad knees, backs, shoulders, necks, etc are quite common. Unfortunately, the scope of this booklet cannot address each individual's situation. Also, some individuals may really want to strengthen or improve a certain body part.

I will outline some sample workouts to give ideas on how to include these exercises along with the others. I suggest you try all of the exercises within your capabilities over time. Then, work the ones that seem to help you the most into your weekly record. If you commit to these exercises and the eating lifestyle system, give it your all and stick with it, I am confident you will see your entire body improve in all areas. Having said that, feel free to e-mail me at *fitfooddude@aol.com* with any questions you may have regarding various exercises. Perhaps I can design and send you an exercise(s) to meet your specific need.

These exercises are outlined by body part or individual muscles. Unlike the previous exercises, these are all *single joint* exercises and target a single muscle group directly. Also, unlike the previous exercises, I recommend you perform each of these exercises just once. Obviously, you can mix it up as you like, but I would simply focus on getting the most out of each movement, and one set will be plenty. The important thing will be for you to *keep* doing them week in and week out. Rome, as they say, was not built in a day. The exercises are as follows:

TRICEPS

One question I often get at seminars is "how do I get rid of my wings?" That is, the excess flab that seems to collect itself around the backs of the upper arms. The general answer, as always, is by adding muscle to your entire body *and* reducing excess body fat from your entire body. The following exercises can help improve the strength, function, and appearance of the upper arms.

Triceps extension:

Function: To strengthen and improve the muscles at the back of the upper arm.
Muscle: Three headed triceps that extends the upper arm.
Resistance: 10-15

1) Stand or sit in a chair or straddling a bench, with a leg on either side.
2) Hold a dumbbell (or dumbbells) overhead with both hands, palms facing up & inward.
3) Inhale while slowly lowering the dumbbell behind your head until your forearms come in contact with your biceps.
4) Keep your head up, back straight and **hold your elbows *in close to your head.***
5) Exhale and extend your elbows until your arms are straight.
6) Make sure the motion is completely controlled, no jerking or excessive straining.

* Can be done one arm at a time, or with two dumbbells at the same time.

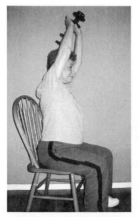 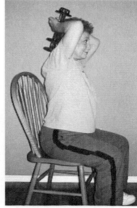

Triceps kickback

Function: To strengthen and develop the triceps muscle (back of upper arm)
Muscles: Triceps (Back of upper arm)
Repetitions: 10-15

1) Lean over the bench, putting your left knee and left palm on the bench top.
2) With your right hand grip the dumbbell, palm facing in. Your upper back and right arm should be parallel to the bench.
3) Hold your elbow in tight to your side and straighten your elbow so that your entire arm becomes parallel to the floor, palm facing in or up.
4) Hold for a second, and then slowly return.
5) Remember to keep your elbow fixed during the entire motion. Repeat with your left arm.

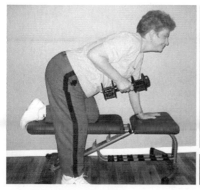
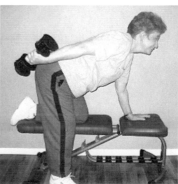

Triceps Push-up

Function: Strengthens/improves back of upper arms
Muscle: Triceps (three headed muscle that extends the upper arm)
Repetitions: 10-15

1) Using a sturdy bench or chair, sit on the edge of the bench or chair with your feet extended in front of you, knees slightly bent.
2) Grasp the edge of the bench, palms facing back, hands in close to body. Lift your buttocks off the bench.
3) Slowly lower your body until you feel a comfortable stretch in your upper arms.
4) Hold for a second then slowly push up to starting position.
5) Remember to keep your back straight and body close to the bench throughout the movement.

* Do not go any lower than the picture indicates. Upper arms should be parallel to the floor. This exercise can be made more challenging by completely straightening the legs or elevating feet by placing them on a stool, chair, etc.

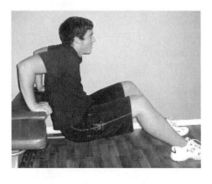

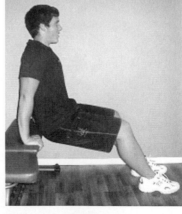

BICEPS

These exercises do more than just create good-looking, stronger biceps. The development of these muscles aid in lifting everyday objects and help to prevent injury to elbows, tendons and ligaments of the forearm.

Standing Curl

Function: To strengthen and improve the upper arms, elbow and forearms.
Muscles: The two-headed biceps and forearm flexors
Repetitions: 10-15

1) Stand upright, knees slightly bent, and feet comfortably spaced apart.
2) With the dumbbells at sides, palms facing in, begin to lift both weights up toward the shoulders, keeping your elbows fixed.
3) As you raise the weight, turn the palms up.
4) Once in the upper position, hold for a second, and then slowly lower the dumbbells back down until your arms are fully extended, palms facing in.

* You can alternate arms for a variation.

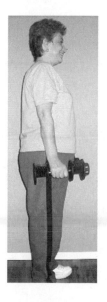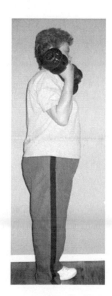

Seated incline curl

Function: Strengthens and improves upper arm and forearms
Muscles: Biceps and forearm flexors
Repetitions: 10-15

1) Sit on incline bench, dumbbells at arms length, palms in.
2) Begin curl with palms in until past thighs, and then turn palms up for remainder of curl to shoulder height.
3) Keep palms up while lowering until past upper thighs, then turn palms in.
4) Keep upper arms and elbows "pinned" close to sides
5) Remember, exhale as you lift, inhale as you lower.

* This exercise is great for stretching and warming up the bicep and elbow joint.

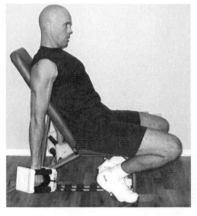 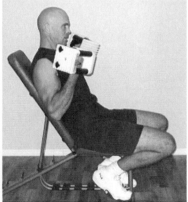

Seated Bicep Curl

Function: Improve strength and functioning of the upper arm and forearm.
Muscles: Biceps and forearm flexors.
Repetitions: 10-15

1) Sit comfortably on a bench or chair, preferably with back supported.
2) Hold dumbbells at your sides with your palms facing inward.
3) Keeping your elbow in a fixed position, lift the dumbbell upward, turning your palm upward as the dumbbell passes your thigh.
4) Bring the dumbbell as close to your shoulder as you can, then lower the dumbbell turning your palm inward as the dumbbell passes your thigh again.
5) Make sure your motions are slow and controlled; do not use momentum to perform this exercise.

* A good variation on this exercise is to alternate arms by lifting and lowering one dumbbell, then the other in a rhythmic manner.

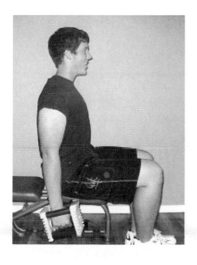 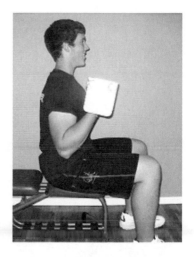

SHOULDERS, NECK & ROTATOR CUFF

Many of us have issues with bad posture & weakness in the shoulder girdle and neck area. These four exercises can help to improve these issues.

Standing lateral (side) raise:

Function: Improves strength and health of shoulder muscles and joint
Muscles: Primarily the side portion of the deltoids (shoulder). Also affects the front and rear parts of this muscle group.
Repetitions: 12-18

1) Stand with feet spaced comfortably apart, bend knees slightly.
2) Holding the dumbbells at your sides, begin to lift them away from your body in an upward and outward motion.
3) Bring your arms up until they reach shoulder level. Do not go above ear level, palms are facing the floor, with thumb a little lower than the rest of the hand.
4) Hold this position for a moment, slowly lower to beginning position.

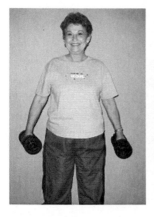 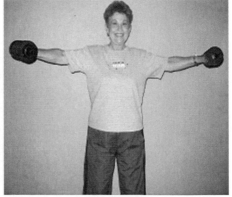

Rotator cuff raise

Function: Improves strength and functioning of the small muscles in the shoulder girdle. These muscles help to "hold" the shoulder together and prevent injury.
Muscles: Upper trapezius, brachialis, levator scapulae, posterior deltoids, rhomboids
Repetitions: 15-25

1) Sit on a bench or the floor, with right leg bent at knee, foot flat on the surface.
2) Holding a light dumbbell in hand, place your right elbow comfortably on your right knee. Your elbow should be a few inches below your shoulder joint.
3) To start, your hand is extended downward, palms facing down. Slowly (4 seconds) raise dumbbell upward in a semi-circle, until dumbbell is straight above kneecap. Do not take dumbbell past this point.
4) Now, slowly lower the dumbbell back to the start. Repeat for desired reps, then switch to the other arm.

* This is a terrific exercise for a strong, functioning and healthy shoulder girdle.

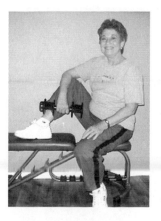 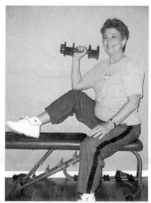

Alternating Shoulder Shrug

Function: Improves posture, health, functioning and strength of the entire shoulder and neck region.

Muscles: Primarily the Trapezius. (Muscles that run from the base of your neck, out to your shoulders, and the upper middle back.

Repetitions: 10-15

This is a simple exercise that many people really like. It just plain "feels good" and helps to work the kinks out of the neck and shoulder regions while improving your health and appearance.

1) Stand straight, chest out and shoulders back, knees slightly bent, holding a dumbbell at your sides.

2) Now, keeping your arm straight, lift one shoulder as high as possible. Imagine you are going to touch your shoulder to your ear. Hold at the top position for one second, and slowly (4 sec) lower the weight.

3) Repeat with the upper arm. That is one rep. Continue on for the correct amount of reps.

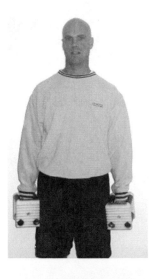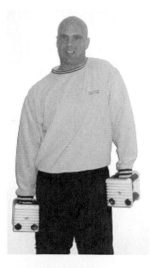

Neck Extension

Function: To improve the strength and health of the neck extensor muscles.

Muscles: Neck extensors. (Used to lift the head up and down).

Repetitions: 8-10

Many people neglect the neck muscles, and that can be a mistake. Do not worry about getting a big neck. The muscles in this area help regulate feelings of stress and impact the nervous system pathways. If you have any issues with your neck, include this exercise in your routine as one of your ten. Take it slowly and breathe deeply!

1) Sit comfortably on a chair, with your body upright and back straight.
2) Clasp your hands comfortably behind your head.
3) Now, *gently* and slowly pull down on your head, while slightly resisting upwards against your hands with your head. You should be able to slowly and steadily move your head downwards. You should feel a pleasant stretch and "burn" in your neck muscles.
4) Stop short of your chin touching your chest. You do not want to yank or force your neck/head at all.
5) Next, slowly begin lifting your head (a 4 second count), this time resisting against your hands. Again, slow and steady. Once back at the starting point, continue on for 8-10 reps.

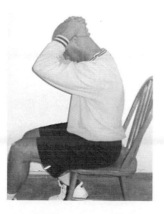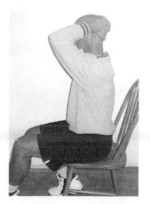

LOWER BODY SINGLE JOINT

Side hip raise

Function: To improve strength and function of hip joint and muscles
Muscles: Gluteus maximus, gluteus minimus, lower back, hip abduction
Repetition: 8-10

1) Stand beside a chair or other sturdy object. Hold onto it lightly. Shift your body weight so that your left leg supports you. Your left knee should be straight (or slightly bent), but not locked. Keep your right toe pointing forward.

2) Slowly lift your leg out to the side, aiming to get your foot 5-8 inches off the ground. Try to keep toes pointed forward and slightly downward. Pause at the top.

3) Slowly lower the foot to the beginning position. Keep going with this leg until you have completed the recommended reps.

Keep your torso upright as possible, avoid leaning to the side. Do not worry too much about how high you lift your foot. Focus on keeping body straight, and focus on the movement in your hip muscles. Once this becomes easier, it will be time to add ankle weights. These can be found in most sporting goods stores or at a website recommended in the back of the book. Start with very light weights and progress.

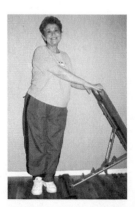 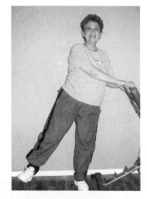

Standing leg curl

Function: to flex the hamstring (upper back of thigh, also known as the "thigh biceps".
Muscle: Hamstrings and lower gluteus.
Repetition: 8-20

1) Stand behind a bench or chair, holding on for support.
2) Feet are together, toes pointing forward. Shift your weight onto your left leg.
3) Now lift your right foot in a semi-circle, until your thigh and lower leg form a ninety-degree angle. Your toes should point straight down.
4) Pause momentarily, and then slowly lower your right foot until only the toes of that foot touch the floor. Continue on until recommended reps are done, then switch to the other leg.

   o   Remember to exhale as you lift, inhale as you lower
   o   Lean only slightly forward, and maintain erect posture.

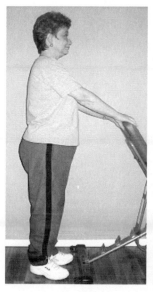 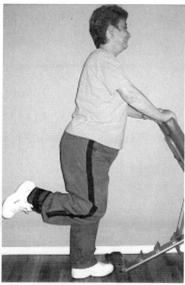

Leg extension

Function: To improve muscles of front thigh, functioning and health of knee joint.
Muscles: Front of upper thigh, especially right above knee joint.
Repetitions: 8-20

1) Sit upright on a chair or bench. Your feet should be shoulder width-apart, with your knees directly above them. Place hands, palms down and overlapping under your left lower thigh. This will elevate that foot so that it can raise and lower without being stopped by the floor.

2) Now, slowly raise your left foot in a semi-circle until the knee is as straight as possible. Keep your toes straight up and gently flexed toward the body. Pause briefly, focus on contracting the thigh muscles and feel the pleasant "burn."

3) Slowly lower the leg to the starting position. Complete the recommended reps with this leg, and then switch to the other one.

* You will need ankle weights for this exercise, but doing this twenty times with no weights is a good start until you get them. Focus on flexing the muscles throughout.

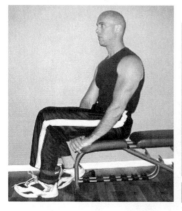 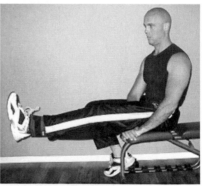

Calf Raise

Function: Improve the muscles and function of the lower leg and ankle.
Muscles: Calf (Gastrocnemius) muscles that extend the foot and toes.
Repetitions: 15-20

1) This exercise requires balance if performed with dumbbells in each hand. If you have problems balancing, use one heavier dumbbell and use the free hand placed against a wall (as pictured).
2) Stand on the floor with your feet spaced comfortably apart.
3) Slowly rise up on your tiptoes, keeping your head level to the ground and back straight. Pause briefly at the top and slowly come back down.
4) * To make this exercise more challenging, try one or all three of the following:

    A) Stand with your toes elevated on a 2" block of wood or similar object.
    B) Stand on one leg, thereby doubling the resistance from body weight.
    C) Try doing this for two minutes straight, no rest, with no weights.

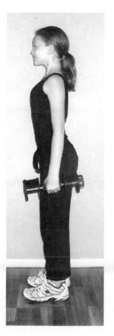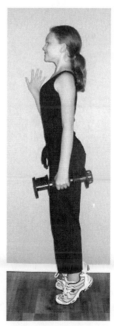

Mountain climbers

This exercise can be used in different ways. It serves to improve the entire lower body by strengthening and increasing your flexibility. By continuing it for several minutes in a row, it can also be used as a cardio/aerobic exercise when you are limited on time or space. I should warn you, if you do this for longer than 10-15 reps, it would make running on a treadmill feel like picking daisies. Start with just 10-15 reps and work into it slowly.

Function: Improves health & function of lower body, legs and back.
Muscles: Thighs, glutes, lower back, shoulders, & heart.
Repetitions: 10-15, eventually up to fifty.

Begin in a hurdles stance. That is both hands on the floor in front of you, looking forward and back flat. Bring your right knee forward until it is directly under your chest. Your knee should be more toward the middle of your body versus the outside.

Now, kick your right foot all the way back while simultaneously bringing your left knee forward to under your chest. Next, kick or extend your left foot backwards to the starting point. That is one rep. Breathe out as you kick back; breathe in as you bring your knees forward.

This may be a bit awkward and quite challenging at first. It is basically running in place while in a sprint position. I encourage you to stick with it though, taking it slow. It will keep you young at heart, if nothing else!

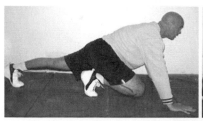 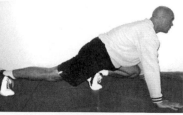

LOWER BACK

Many people have difficulties with their lower backs. This is often due to a deconditioned body, excessive body fat, and weak muscles, especially of the abdomen, lower back, gluteus, and thigh muscles. I would recommend that you follow the strength-training program outlined to improve the health and functioning of your *entire* body. As you do and improve your eating, the health of your back will improve as well. Still, I would like to show you two exercises that have helped the backs of others (including mine!). These exercises can improve the strength and flexibility of the upper and lower back and spinal column. The second one requires the use of an exercise ball. Be sure you get the right size ball for your body size, and one that is strong and durable. They can be purchased at high quality fitness stores or on the Internet at *www.chekinstitute.com.*

HALF BRIDGE

Function: Improve the health and function of the lower back and glutes.
Muscles: Lower back, glutes (butt), front of upper thighs, abdominal.
Repetitions: 10-20

1) Lie on floor, knees bent, feet flat on the floor.
2) Keep arms straight on floor at side as you lift hips up.
3) Push with your glutes until the body is straight.
4) Hold in top position for a moment, feeling the muscles and stretch.
5) Lower and repeat, exhale up and inhale down.

* This is terrific for the lower back & body.

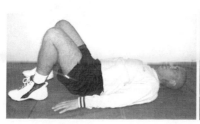 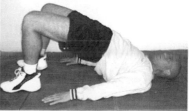

Back Bridge with a ball

Function: To improve strength and flexibility of upper and lower back and abs.
Muscles: Upper and lower back, glutes, abs.
Repetitions: 8-20

1) Clear a spot free of any sharp or hard objects, with a soft surface floor or mat.

2) Sit on exercise ball, with feet firmly anchored or on the floor. Slowly and carefully lay back on the ball, keeping arms folded across the chest. When you feel fully secure, slowly stretch your arms over your head, trying to place your hands on the floor.

3) When you have reached as far as you can, inhale and exhale deeply and relax your body, letting your upper body "hang" to provide a good stretch.

4) Now, using your legs, slowly move your body back and forth lengthwise across the ball, just a few inches each way is all that it takes.

* This should help to loosen the lower back, and increase blood flow to that area. You can do this on your non-weightlifting days. Focus on deep breathing!

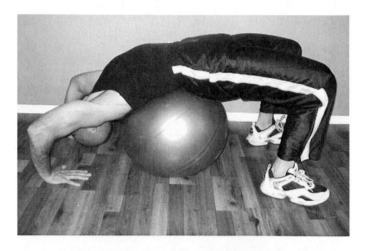

Additional comments on the Knees and Back:

The foundational and assistive exercises outlined above will help to improve these areas tremendously. It is always important to remember that the body is systemic. That is, it is a complete system, where everything depends upon each other component and works together. The first step to relieving problems in these two areas is to strengthen your entire body and reduce/eliminate any extra body fat you are carrying. Until then, only so much improvement can be made. Meanwhile, work harder on improving the muscle groups *around* these two areas. For example, it is well known that back problems are tied to weak abdominals. What is not as well known is that back problems are also related to a weak butt, hamstrings, and upper back. As you strengthen those areas, your back will greatly benefit. Likewise, strengthening your hamstrings, front thighs and butt will help your knees.

What about my abs?

Many people are carrying excessive body fat in this area. Therefore, we see millions of ab rollers and other silly infomercial "six pack making" gadgets sold on TV, modeled by people who have probably NEVER used one to get the well-defined abs they possess. Good abdominal muscle appearance and function are the result of a well-muscled body developed through a consistently active lifestyle that has involved several months if not years of strengthening and cardio exercise in combination with being properly nourished. Proper nourishment means paying closer attention to eating sufficient lean proteins, fresh high fiber whole vegetables and fruits, natural fats, and non-processed, high fiber, complex carbohydrates while reducing overly refined, sweetened, and additive filled foods.

I often do not have students do *any* ab exercises until their body fat has been reduced enough so that their abdominal muscles can be seen. Until then, if a person is breathing properly and doing the major exercises correctly, their abs are getting plenty of work. The best strength exercises for reducing excess abdominal fat are those that involve the larger muscle systems of the body, such as the legs, butt, upper back and chest. Be sure to follow your strength training with proper cardio work, and you will be light years ahead of any AB thing a ma jig. Make it a goal to be able to see your abdominal muscles (don't get neurotic though) and *then* you can start with the crunches. If that seems like an eternity to you, consider waiting at least wait three months. In the meantime, perform the other exercises above with consistency and eat better by following the guidelines suggested in the next section. Remember; be patient, diligent, and disciplined. Most of us didn't get into our current condition overnight! When you are ready to move on to crunches, simply substitute them for one of the accessory exercises, always keeping your total at ten exercises for the day. Or, you can simply perform your crunches on your non-weight training days.

Crunches with feet supported on bench/chair

Function: Improve strength of abdominal area and lower back/spine
Muscles: Abs (Rectus abdominus), neck flexors
Repetitions: 20

1) Lying on your back with your feet hanging over a bench or chair, place your hands so they are lightly touching the sides of your head.

2) Maintain a 90-degree angle between your upper and lower legs, with the small of your lower back pressed into the floor.

3) Using only your abdominal muscles, lift your head and shoulders off the floor. Try to point your chin at the ceiling above, keep your mouth open to avoid holding your breath. Only lift as far as you can without excessive straining. We do not need to lift far on this to make a good impact.

4) Do not use your arms and neck to pull your head forward, let the abs do the work.

5) Once in the upper position, hold for two seconds and then slowly lower yourself back down.

    o   Do not be fooled into thinking that one must do hundreds of these. 20 focused, controlled reps will do wonders if done consistently.

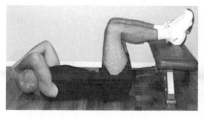 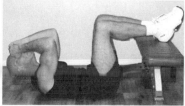

Cardiovascular/Aerobic Exercise

Although cardiovascular/aerobic exercise has been addressed to a degree throughout this book, a little more detailed instruction will now be provided in order to help structure your workout in the most effective method possible. If you are like me, you prefer to keep it simple. This section contains a few formulas' that might scare some of us off. Please, take a few moments to read this section, as these formulas are really quite easy to learn and remember and can help safeguard and improve your life.

The benefits of cardiovascular/aerobic exercise have been widely proclaimed over the past 35 years or so. Cardiovascular/aerobic exercise is defined as exercise that involves moving the large muscle groups of the body for an sustained period of time while taking the heart rate to a higher than resting level. I have used the terms cardiovascular (cardio for short) and aerobic together, because most people consider them to be the same type of activity. The primary profit of cardio/aerobic exercise, as the name depicts, is thought to be to improve the health and functioning of the heart, veins and arteries.

Aerobic means, "with oxygen", but the most significant advantage of this exercise is that when done consistently, it creates additional "aerobic pathways" to the working muscle groups. That is, it builds additional arteries to those muscle groups. Thus, they are able to tap into more blood flow and oxygen when needed, allowing the muscles to perform their tasks more efficiently and for longer periods of time. This is good for the heart and all of the major systems of the body, because there is then less strain placed upon them. Strength training, as you now know, can accomplish much of the same and more.

Nevertheless, cardio and aerobic exercise is incredibly valuable, and is capable of challenging our bodies in a different and needed way that strength training does not always reach. So, if a person wants the best for their lives, they should make it a regular part of their lifestyle. The benefits it offers includes:

A) Increased burning of calories.
B) Reduction of excess body fat when done correctly.
C) Release of endorphins, the "runners" high effect of improved mood and good feelings.
D) Improved health of the heart, lungs, arteries, and entire body.
E) Helps you to relax, feel less stressed, sleep better and feel better.
F) Helps you to sweat, cleansing and removing impurities from the body.
G) Challenges your mental fortitude and self-discipline.
H) Improves your confidence about handling physical tasks and your health future.
I) Improves endurance and stamina of all the major muscle groups and systems of the body.
J) Helps with mental clarity, focus and thinking.
K) Reinforces eating better, not smoking or drinking in excess.
L) Improves flexibility and functioning of joints, tendons and ligaments.
M) Helps to strengthen and build the muscles of the body to a limited degree. Not nearly as much as strength training, but if you have been a couch potato you will see some muscle growth if done correctly.
N) Improves overall health and fitness and will help you to live better and most likely live longer.

As you can see, that is an impressive list. There are in fact numerous additional, more specific benefits for our lives from cardio work, but the list above sums it up. Nonetheless, as you know, cardio ALONE is not the most effective type of exercise for the majority of Americans to reach their healthiness goals. Rather, when it is *combined* with muscle building exercise is when it can truly have a positive impact. Yet, for those who are doing cardio/aerobic exercise, most do it incorrectly. That is, if they are seriously seeking the best way to become lean, fit, strong and healthy. The three primary mistakes made with cardio/aerobic exercise are:

I)   Doing ONLY cardio/aerobic exercise. "I use my treadmill everyday!"
II) Doing cardio/aerobic exercise for too long and at too low of an intensity level.
III) Doing cardio/aerobic exercise BEFORE strength training.

So what should you do? You have two options to choose from. The first option is best, but both will work. Option # 1 is *IMMEDIATELY* after your strength training session; perform 12-15 minutes of higher intensity cardio/aerobic exercise. The reason for this is that if you have strength trained correctly, your metabolism will be sky high. By doing your cardio/aerobic right after strength training, you will be taking advantage of your optimal metabolism and fat-burning zone. An added advantage is that this method saves time, as you can now take the next day off from exercising, which allows your muscles to grow and your body to recuperate. This is particularly important for those who are newer to exercising or especially pressed for time (most of us).

Option # 2 is to perform your cardio/aerobic on your non-strength training days. For example, if you weight train on Mon-Wed-Fri, you could do "cardio" on Tues-Thurs-Sat. This is what many other exercise books suggest, and it is an effective alternative. If you choose this method, however, perform 20 minutes of cardio, versus 12-15. There is no need to go past 20 minutes. If you perform this exercise with the correct intensity, I can assure you, 20 minutes will be plenty! More will be explained about that in a moment.

When cardio/aerobic exercise first became popular, jogging was the primary method used. Over the years, running, "power walking", treadmills, aerobics classes, stationary bikes, aerobic kickboxing, spinning, rowing and so on have grown in popularity as methods to engage in cardio/aerobic exercise. Most any of these methods will be fine. My own preferences include jogging, interval hill sprints or a recumbent bike on days when the weather is particularly nasty. Choose from one of the above activities or any that allows you to take your heart rate to a moderate to intense level for 12-20 minutes.

How hard should I work at my cardio exercise?

Part of the answer to the above will depend upon your current physical condition. If you have not been exercising, please work into this progressively. In fact, for some of you, walking at a brisk pace may be a good starting point. We must keep things in perspective. If you have been sedentary, the fact that you are now becoming active is a terrific beginning. When considering how hard to push yourself as you progress with this type of exercise, there are three methods to choose from to insure safety and results.

Target heart zone

The first, and perhaps most widely known, is the target heart zone. The idea behind this method is to determine a "zone" of heart beat which would be safe and effective for an individual, and which they could maintain for 12-20 minutes. The standard formula for establishing this is as follows:

A)   Determine your maximum heart rate (MHR) by subtracting your age from 220. For example, I am currently 45. So, 220-45 = 175. 175 is my recommended maximum heart rate (MHR).

B)   Determine your correct training zone. It is recommended that we perform our cardio exercise at between 50-90 % of our MHR. If you are de-conditioned or new to exercise, it is best to stay near the 50% effort level at first. So, in my case that would mean 175 (My max heart rate) x .50 = 87.5. Thus, for starters my target heart zone (THZ) is about 88 beats per minute. From there I will want to continually progress to between 60-80 % on a consistent basis.

How can you determine what your heart rate is while exercising? While there are manual methods for doing so, most are cumbersome and complicated. So if you want to know what heart rate you are at while performing your cardio, simply purchase a heart rate monitor. The best ones I have seen are like wristwatches that you wear while exercising that give you an instant readout. These can be purchased at most sporting goods stores or online at *www.polarusa.com*. The Polar models are more expensive, yet excellent quality. The "Polar F1" retails for about $60.00 and is great for most of us.

Borg Rating of Perceived Exertion

A second method to monitor and measure how hard you are working during cardio exercise is known as the, "Borg Rating of Perceived Exertion Scale". Gunnar Borg developed it around 1970. This is a simple practical method that anyone can do. Perceived exertion is how hard you feel like your body is working. It is based on the physical sensations a person experiences during physical activity, including increased heart rate, breathing, sweating and muscle fatigue. Although this is a subjective (guessing!) measure, according to Borg, a person's exertion rating can provide a fairly good estimate of the actual heart rate during exercise.

Trainers have concluded that ratings of 12-14 on the Borg scale show that exercise is being performed at a moderate level of intensity. As you exercise, use the Borg Scale below to assign numbers to how you feel. Self-monitoring how hard your body is working can help you adjust the intensity of the activity by speeding up or slowing down your movements. Through experience of monitoring how your body feels, it will become easier to know when to adjust your intensity. For example, a walker who wants to engage in moderate-intense activity would aim for a Borg Scale level of "somewhat hard" (12-14). If he describes his muscle fatigue and breathing as "very light" (9 on the Borg Scale) he would want to increase his intensity. Likewise, if he felt his exertion was "extremely hard" (19 on the Borg Scale) he would need to slow down his movements to achieve the moderate-intensity range.

Instructions for Borg Rating of Perceived Exertion (RPE) Scale

While exercising, rate your perceived exertion. This feeling should reflect how heavy and strenuous the exercise feels to you, combining all sensations and feelings of physical stress effort and fatigue. Do not concern yourself with any one factor such as leg pain or shortness of breath, but try to focus on your total feeling of exertion.

Look at the rating scale while you are exercising. It will only be necessary for you to do this until you are familiar with the scale. The scale ranges from 6-20, where 6 means "no exertion at all" and 20 means "maximal exertion". Choose the number below that best describes your level of exertion. This will give you a good idea of the intensity level of your cardio exercise, and you can use this information to speed up or slow down to reach your preferred range.

Try to estimate your feeling of exertion as accurately as possible, without thinking about what the actual physical load is. Your own feeling of effort and exertion is important, not how it compares to other people. Look at the scales and the descriptions and then state a number.

6 No exertion at all	14
7-8 Extremely light	15 Hard (Heavy)
9 Very light	16
10	17 Very hard
11 Light	18
12	19 Extremely hard
13 Somewhat hard	20 Maximal exertion

9 Corresponds to "very light" exercise. For a healthy person, it is like walking slowly at his or her own pace for some minutes.

13 on the scale is "somewhat hard" exercise, but it still feels ok to continue.

17 "Very hard" is very strenuous. A healthy person can still go on, but he or she really has to push him or herself. It feels very hard (challenging), and the person is very tired.

19 This is an extremely strenuous exercise level. For most people, this is the most strenuous exercise they have ever experienced.

The talk test

The Berg Scale is good in that it simply takes a little time to become familiar with and requires no technical knowledge or equipment. To simplify things even further, apply the "talk" test. As you are performing your cardio exercise, imagine that you are having a conversation with someone. If you are able to talk and converse as normal, without pause to catch a breath, you are likely not working hard enough. If, on the opposite end, you are unable to talk at all while exercising, you may be working at too high of an intensity level. The goal is to be able to converse some, but having to pause between sentences now and then to catch your breath.

Interval training

This method can be used in combination with either of the above. It is useful in adding variety to your cardio workouts and good for speeding up your metabolism while preserving your life-protecting coat of muscle. This method is **not** for a person who is in poor condition or new to exercise. After they have been training a while, they could work into it. There are a few ways in which to use this type of training, but the simplest is as follows. You will need a stopwatch or timer of some sort.

After you have performed your strength-training workout, it is time for your 12 minutes of cardio. With the interval method, you would begin the first thirty seconds at a light or 50% maximum heart rate (MHR) effort. Then, the next thirty seconds you would step up the intensity a bit, say to "somewhat hard" or 60 % MHR. The next thirty seconds would be taken back to the 50 % MHR, and then the next thirty seconds back up to perhaps a higher level of effort, say 65-

70 % MHR or "hard" level. The idea is basically to "zigzag" your efforts up, down, up, down. It is effective and a method you will eventually want to incorporate into your cardio program. One of the other reasons I like this method is that it allows you to progressively test yourself as to how high of an intensity level you can safely go for a short period of time. Try it, you will like it!

One hour recommendation?

For decades the "experts" have been recommending 30 minutes of exercise per day. Now that our nation has reached epidemic obesity levels and shockingly poor health, the latest recommendation has been increased to one hour. This makes no sense for several reasons. First off, if people aren't going to exercise for thirty minutes, what makes anyone think they will jump into one hour? Second, several studies have shown that more intense exercise yields greater results and benefits than lower intensity exercise. The fact is, a person can either work harder or work longer, but they cannot do both.

Thus, in our quest for the best, it is most excellent to eventually work a little harder, smarter and for a shorter period of time. Most of us are time challenged. If you performed the weight lifting workouts in this book, three days a week for thirty minutes followed by 12-15 minutes of appropriate intensity cardio work, that would add up to 135 exercise minutes in a week. You could, of course do more, but it is truly not needed, especially for the first year or so of taking up this lifestyle.

The fact is, if everyone in the country did the above workout schedule, ate closer to the food guidelines coming up in the next chapters, did not drink alcoholic beverages in excess or smoke, we would see unfathomable improvements in our nations fitness. I don't like the one-hour recommendation because it is not specific enough and discourages the already discouraged. Having said that, we all need to get more active, obviously. I am convinced that as you or others become more fit, strong, and healthy, becoming more active for longer periods of time will naturally follow as a sensible way of life.

On the following pages are forms and examples of possible workouts you could follow. One could design their own workout or follow the workouts as outlined, or make substitutions for exercises that may not currently be suitable to you. And, please do not hesitate or be shy about e-mailing me if you are unsure of anything I have outlined. I am dedicated to the success of each and every person who has invested in this book. My e-mail is fitfooddude@aol.com.

Week at a Glance Workout Schedule

Monday-Wednesday-Friday:
Strength-training for 25-30 minutes, followed by 12-15 minutes of appropriate intensity "cardio" work. As stated, one could do their cardio for 20 minutes on Tues, Thurs & Saturday instead of right after their strength training.

Tuesday-Thursday-Saturday:
Either no exercise, or simply do one set each of pushups (as many as possible), deep knee bends (AMAP), and crunches or bridges. Many students *want* to exercise on their non-weight lifting days, sometimes for nothing more than to shake the cobwebs, get the heart pumping, de-stiffen the joints and muscles and stay in the activity habit. If you are doing your cardio on non-weight lifting days and are especially ambitious, you could combine the bodyweight exercises with the cardio.

The bodyweight only exercises can be done two days in a row, as they do not tend to break down the muscle fibers to the same degree as weight lifting does. Again, if the ones I've listed are too challenging at this point, find ones more suitable for now. Just remember to include a major upper and lower body exercise and one for your mid-section (lower back and/or abdominal muscles).

Sunday:
Day of rest

Blank workout scoreboard

Exercise:	Date:	Date:	Date:	Date:	Date:	Date:
Upper Body *PUSH:*	wt. / reps					
Upper Body *PUSH:*						
Upper Body *PULL:*						
Upper Body *PULL:*						
Lower Body:						
Lower Body:						
Your choice						
Your choice						
Your choice						
Your choice						

For additional chart samples to
fit your needs go to:
www.fitfooddude.com

On the road again workout

A question frequently received is, "how can I continue working out when I travel?" The answer is uncomplicated. Prepare ahead. I travel frequently, and have three approaches to making sure I can train in some fashion, literally no matter where I go. I can either train in a local gym; a hotel where I might be staying or plan on doing body weight only exercises in my hotel room, at the campground, etc.

If, for example, I know I am going to Indianapolis, Indiana and will be staying at the downtown Hyatt, I will call ahead to ask if they have a fitness center. Over the years I have found that many so-called "fitness centers" at hotels are nothing more than a few treadmills or cardio only equipment. That of course, is not a true fitness center. So, I always ask, "do you have serious strength training equipment, including weights." The number of hotels with real weights in their exercise rooms is growing, but it is still about 50/50. If they do have weights or a decent strength-training machine, the problem is handled.

If not, I will ask the concierge if there is a good health club nearby, and if so, for their phone number. Then of course, I call the gym for more information on their facilities and their daily rate for out-of town guests. Sometimes their daily fees are high, but this is something I am committed to, and if the gym is not far from where I am staying, I may "exercise" this option.

A third option, and one I choose more and more often, is to work out in a room or out doors wherever I am staying. In this case, a routine of bodyweight only exercises and a brief (12-15 minutes) cardio/aerobic routine are used. For example, this summer we spent a week visiting my mother and staying at her home. Each morning I would get up a few minutes earlier than everyone else, and proceed to the basement. There, I performed a 15-minute workout of some form of pushups (regular or chair) for the upper body "push" muscle system, deep knee bends (lunges or flat footed squats are great too!) to train the legs and lower body, crunches for the ABS and lower back and bridging for the upper back and entire body. After that I either went for a jog/run or did mountain climbers. Mountain climbers are a great way to do cardio, and can be done indoors with little room. The technique and instructions for doing them are on page 186. These are not for the faint of heart, however.

Another, perhaps more viable option for getting your cardio, especially at a hotel, is simply stair climbing. Most hotels have at least one set of stairs. Depending upon your fitness level, you could simply climb stairs for 12-20 minutes at a quick pace. Make a trip up the stairs, then descend the stairs at a safe but lively pace, and start back up. If you are more fit, take two steps at a time, and for the advanced, try sprinting up the stairs two steps at a time or running up the stairs as fast as you can, one step at a time. Be sure your shoes are non-slip, and watch out for traffic! In fact, if you have stairs close to your home, you may want to make stair climbing a regular part of your weekly workout. It is an awesome conditioner.

As you can see, there are no excuses for not working out while traveling. And, my experience has been that it helps overcome jet-lag and any substandard foods you may have indulged in. Also, it really helps to build confidence and energy, knowing that you have the self-discipline to adapt to different environments, no matter where you go.

Measurements

These are of course, optional. Measurements can help to encourage us, when they are used properly and kept in perspective. My suggestion is to take them, and then take them again, every 30 days. Until then put them in a safe place, forget about them and get to work on the workouts and eating better. After one month, take them again, and note your progress, and any adjustments you may want to make in your workout intensity, exercises, etc. Always remember though, the most important measurement is the fact that you are involved in a progressive fitness lifestyle. That is immeasurably the most important thing, more than any number we can read.

To do all the desired measurements you will need a reliable bodyweight scale, measuring tape, and body-fat calipers. Excellent and inexpensive calipers and measuring tapes can be purchased online at accufitness.com or fitfooddude.com. Measurements should be taken before training and after three months. You should measure your:

- Bodyweight
- Neck
- Chest
- Right upper arm
- Waist (at belly button)
- Right thigh, middle
- Right calf

Body fat & lean mass skin folds

I am a huge fan of measuring body fat. Earlier chapters dealt with the subject of throwing away your scale. Scales can be helpful in establishing a baseline from which to work. The problem, as discussed, is that scales do not measure what really matters, and that is body composition. Body composition, for our purposes, really involves only two things. They are, excess body fat and lean mass (primarily muscle). Scales do not measure these things. An additional problem with a scale is that when a person takes up a muscle adding lifestyle, they will initially sometimes ADD bodyweight. Then, they get on the scale and freak out when they see their bodyweight increasing, and think this isn't "working" for them. The truth is that what is happening is actually good and what we want. As they are adding muscle, though their bodyweight is increasing, so is their metabolism, which in turn behaves like Pac-Man and gradually helps to gobble up our excess body fat.

The fact is, if you are going to measure body fat versus lean mass (muscle) it is best to get a set of body fat calipers. I have referenced above the ones I recommend. They are called "Accumeasures" and come from a company called Accufitness. I offer them on my website for a few bucks cheaper than the company, but the company's website has other cool stuff. Again, it is *www.accufitness*. Please just tell them I sent you! The calipers come with a small instruction book. The book details how best to determine your ideal body weight and a very easy method to measure excess body fat. All that is required is a quick skin fold measurement above the right hipbone. I don't agree wholeheartedly with their nutrition guidelines, but the rest of the info is great. The calipers generally range from $17-20, which is quite a bargain for information that could save your life. There are numerous other ways to measure body fat, yet none are really more accurate and most are more expensive and impractical for a good number of us.

The scale below offers guidelines for body-fat percentage. I have seen numerous such scales with different descriptions of the body fat ranges. This one is one of the best I've spotted. Please keep in mind that no measurement is entirely accurate. I have witnessed some people become a bit neurotic and compulsive in their desire to attain the "ideal" body fat percentage. Remember, the goal is to *progressively* get better and healthier, not add another mental stressor to our lives. With that in mind, the following guidelines can be helpful in giving us a reasonable goal to shoot for:

Body Fat Percentage

Essential
- Women: 10-12% fat
- Men 2-4% fat

Athletes
- Women: 14-20% fat
- Men 6-13% fat

Fitness
- **Women: 12-24% fat**
- **Men 14-17% fat**

Acceptable
- Women: 25-31% fat
- Men 18-25% fat

Obese
- Women: 32% fat and higher
- Men 25% fat++

The goal for most of us is to be in the fitness range. Some body fat is needed by all of us, as depicted in the "essential" range. Just as in having too much body fat can be dangerous, likewise having too little (the essential range) is not suggested either.

What is a Workout?

A workout is 25% perspiration and 75% determination. Stated another way, it is one part physical exertion and three parts self-discipline. Doing it is enjoyable when it becomes habit.

A workout makes you better today than you were yesterday. It strengthens the body, relaxes the mind and toughens the spirit. When you work out regularly, your problems diminish and your confidence grows.

A workout is a personal triumph over laziness and procrastination. It is a badge of a winner—the mark of an organized, goal-oriented person who has taken charge of his or her destiny.

A workout is a wise use of time and an investment in excellence. It is a way of preparing for life's challenges and proving to yourself that you have what it takes to do what is necessary. A workout is a key that helps unlock the door to opportunity and success. Hidden within each of us is an extraordinary force. Physical and mental fitness are triggers that can help to release it.

A workout is a form of rebirth. When you finish a good workout, you don't simply feel better—you feel better about yourself!

www.fitfooddude.com

Section VI

Food and Nutrition Made

Simple and Sane

*Why all you need to succeed can be
learned from babies, my mother,
and those who lived off of
the fruited plain.*

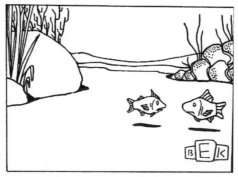

"Now they're saying shiny things attached to hooks are bad for you."

Chapter 17

Thoroughbreds Don't Eat Twinkies

It used to be said that politics and religion were topics to be avoided in a conversation unless you were looking for a fight or at least a heated argument. In recent years, food seems to have joined the field of religion and politics. More specifically, the relationships of food, eating and staying lean and healthy have become topics of hot debate. At the same time, hundreds of authors and some supposed experts are making millions of dollars offering their solutions. Ironically, each of these sources states they have the answer for you. So it is with just a little trepidation that I tread into this food territory. My objective is to add degree of simplicity and saneness into the arena, in the hopes of helping those who may have become dazed and confused by all of the food and nutrition madness.

But one thing is for sure. Food and eating is something that is near and dear to us. All of us enjoy eating and get much pleasure from the experience. A good meal is a good thing. Unfortunately though, for some, food has almost become a substitute for other things that are supposed to meet our emotional needs. For many, food has become the great comforter, which takes away pain, relieves boredom, and gives us the illusion of reducing stress. Indeed, it has been said that America's number one anti-anxiety medication is . . . food.

A good meal certainly brings comfort to our taste buds, satisfies our stomach and meets the physiological needs of the body, but we all know that no food is capable of meeting the needs of our emotions and soul. Still, try taking away a person's favorite comfort food, and you may find that some people have very strong emotional attachments to their food. I know this from personal experience as a trainer. I have suggested to fully-grown men that they consider reducing a certain food from their menu and it nearly reduces them to tears! Yes, I'm exaggerating a bit, but not much.

Soon, I will address the more popular "diets" that are all over the media these days as well as the established food guide pyramid. First, however, I would like to outline the, "Fit Food Formula." It is built on 21 basic principles. **IT IS NOT A DIET, BUT A LIFESTYLE!** It is also not magic. Making healthy food choices are not all that complicated so you may find some overlap with current "diet" trends. Still, there are some basic, unique principles you will learn that when utilized in conjunction with strength training and briefer, higher intensity cardio, deliver definite success. I know from past experience there will be a few critics of the "formula", and I will address those criticisms throughout the next few chapters. Let me say up front, the formula allows for eating a healthy balance of all foods, excludes no foods groups, provides for all essential nutrients and still allows you to enjoy your favorite "junk" food now and then.

Sometimes I joke about eating "for function, not flavor". Most do the opposite and eat almost solely for flavor, which is nearly as ridiculous as eating solely for function. The Fit Food Formula provides a balance. It is flexible and requires less work than most any other eating "scheme" available. And never fear, you will still get to enjoy great food. I love to eat good food as much as anyone. That is one of the reasons I was attracted to the food business! You may need to modify some of your favorites a bit, or have them less often, but long-term deprivation of foods we really enjoy doesn't work very well. You also won't go hungry to the point of stomach growling or hunger pains. In fact, for some of you, you may find yourself eating more foods than ever before.

As these principles are outlined, the initial focus will be on function. It is important for you to know *why* you are doing certain things, and how they work in conjunction with your body. Later on, we will discuss *how* to implement these principles into our eating habits that will last a lifetime. Before we break down the principles in greater detail, however, lets take a summary look at them. These principles are the best in existence for 99 people out of 100 to become as fit, dynamically healthy, and lean as is humanly possible.

Some have commented that these 21 principles are too much, that they are a bit overwhelming and may scare people off. A professor in nutrition told me that there is no way anyone will *ever* do all these things. My response to her was that I hope to bring out the best in myself and in other people. One of the keys to doing that is to *expect* the best. So when someone comes to me for training, or sits in my audience at a conference, I imagine that they are paying me one million dollars to hear what I have to say. It is my responsibility to give them the best and all that I know and believe will help them achieve the most magnificent results possible. What they choose to do with the 21 principles is up to them. Some may choose to implement these principles into their lives all at once, others little by little. If they choose to use only a few, they will still be much better for it. If they want to walk away and look for something easier, that is also their choice. My job is to expect and deliver the best. So you are getting all 21 principles.

After we cover the 21 basics, we will go into a little more detail on each one to clarify precisely what we are talking about. There are a few differences I hope you will notice right away in these principles. They are not just about food. The first six principles are the pillars, the rest are the bricks. **Master the first six principles first.** They are the most crucial, and hold everything together.

Fit Food Dude's Proven 21 "Pillars and Bricks" to Permanently Becoming a Lean, Fat-Incinerating, Anti-Aging, Wellness Machine!

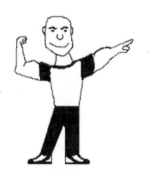

The Pillars

1) **Have a written, specific goal.** Stated in positive terms of how you want to improve your healthiness. Without a goal, we are simply wishing into the wind. Commit it to paper, and your objective will have a superior chance of becoming reality versus a daydream or vapor.

2) **Workout consistently and correctly.** If you are not committed to exercising consistently and correctly, there is really no sense in reading any further.

3) **Strength train first, cardio second.** You *must* strength train if you want the best for yourself. Do aerobic or adjunct exercise as well, but **after** you strength train.

4) **Eat breakfast within 15-20 minutes of waking up.** Otherwise, call it brunch and watch your metabolism slow down to a barely perceptible crawl.

5) **Eat 5-8 smaller (6 is best), equally sized meals per day, every 2-3.5 hours.** Our new definition of a meal is *any* time we put *any* food in our mouth.

6) **Eat *MORE* real, fresh food.** This includes lean proteins, fresh high fiber vegetables, fruits, adequate (not excessive!) natural fats, and a moderate amount of *high fiber, unaltered, complex*

carbohydrates. Think of foods that you can pick, pull from the ground, milk or catch.

The Bricks

7) **Keep records of food intake and workouts.** Those who have the best chance of winning are those who know the score. Keep a daily journal of what and when you eat and drink. Likewise, write down exercise achievements such as weight used, times lifted, distance walked, etc. Feedback is the breakfast of champions!

8) **Eliminate the words "dieting, diet and/or losing weight" from your vocabulary forever!!** To "diet" alone is a foolish and unhealthy behavior.

9) **Establish in your mind more positive and productive healthiness behaviors.** Focus on transforming body composition by restoring lost muscle and reducing excess body fat. This requires activity/exercise that builds or maintains lean body mass (muscle & bone), eating well, sleeping enough and reducing chronic harmful stress.

10) **Establish a "junk food session".** This is a 1-3 hour period each week (once a week!) to indulge *a little.* Mine is almost always Friday night. Pizza, oven baked fries and ice cream are my favorites!

11) **Invest in a good Igloo cooler with ice packs.** This can be your body's best friend. You wouldn't drive your car without gas in the tank would you? Always be prepared.

12) **Reduce or eliminate** all carbs (except green fibrous vegetables) the **last one or two** meals before bedtime. Do not eat or drink anything (except water) after 8:00 pm. (Preferably 7:00)

13) **Determine your approximate calorie target per day.** You will learn how to do this and it does not have to be perfect. But if you have no clue, that spells less health for you.

14) **Determine your approximate calorie target per meal.** Again, perfection is not the goal. Awareness of how much your body really needs per "feeding" is.

15) **Watch out for "brain suckers".** These include the age-old stimulants and addictive habits of alcohol, caffeine, sugar,

fructose, nicotine & artificial sweeteners, etc. Excessive stimulants can cause our energy to expire prematurely. Sometimes permanently.

16) **Don't fall for Supplement heaven.** If you follow the guidelines above, you may not need any supplements. Supplements are *primarily* sold to those who are not willing to work harder at the basics of exercising and eating well. Perhaps take a good vitamin/mineral pill and essential fatty acid oil.

17) **Focus on portions, not servings.** It is better to eat a little fresh broccoli than none at all. We don't need to eat a half-cup of everything to gain some of its benefits.

18) **Learn the basics of protein, fat, and carbohydrates.** Take a few hours and study the fundamentals of protein, fat and carbohydrates. Without knowledge, success is doubtful.

19) **Measure what you can.** Especially at first. If a dish calls for a tablespoon of something, use a tablespoon to measure it out! Little things often make a big difference.

20) **Fill up on fiber.** The combination of lean protein and fiber are the one-two punch to knocking off excess body fat. Colon cancer doesn't sound like much fun either. Keep the pipes clean!

21) **Find a partner, coach, or at least an encourager.** Hook up with someone who will cheer you on, keep you in balance, and kick you in the rear when you need it. Partners improve our success odds by 37%!!

"We know that cholesterol, hypertension and inactivity are proven precursors to many health problems. We also know that it is up to us to make a commitment to do something about it. But my commitment was on and off until I heard you speak at our association's annual conference. Somehow, you peeked the interest of a self-proclaimed skeptic when it comes to conference presenters. You are a true believer in a healthy lifestyle and it shows. Since I heard your interesting and motivational presentation I have taken on a new LIFE STYLE by following your recommendations. For some reason, when you said "trust me, it works," I did. The results have been so astounding both mentally and physically. I would highly recommend

your methods for a refreshing and workable approach to health."
Registered Dietitian, M.S. Nutritional Science

The quote above is from a woman who came to my seminar. She continually challenged me on the validity of my recommendations and claims of how it could work for people. At the time we were simply reviewing the principles outlined above. As I recall, she specifically felt that I was recommending too much protein and too much food. I replied that if a person was following the exercise and active lifestyle suggested, they would be fine following these principles . . . perhaps finer than they have ever been. I assured her that I had been following such a plan for over 20 years, and that my kidneys and everything else were operating just fine. In addition, I know of many other healthy, fit, lean and strong adults who can say the same. Finally, out of exasperation, I simply said, "try it, it works".

To my surprise, I ran into my "challenger" at another conference approximately three months later. She informed me that she had been trying to reach me but could not find my e-mail, etc. It turns out that previous to hearing me speak; her doctor had diagnosed her with high blood pressure and cholesterol. He told her that if she were unable to get it under control, he would have to put her on medications. This 62-year-old woman, with advanced degrees in nutrition, was struggling to get her weight and health under control. She had tried the conventional methods she had been trained in, and had not found the success she was hoping for.

So now, here it was, almost three months later. According to this woman, since hearing me speak, she had lost 20 pounds of excess body fat, her blood pressure and cholesterol had normalized, she was far more active, her husband wanted to thank me personally, and her doctor was marveling at her "miracle" healthiness makeover. This stuff does indeed work, my friend. But perhaps you need a little more detail. For that reason, we will quickly review each principle, and offer a few simple calculations and charts where needed. Then, additional "secrets" to successfully staying lean through eating that are easy to remember and you can live with for a lifetime will be suggested. These principles are not meant to overwhelm you. Sometimes people feel these are "restrictions" designed to rob them of enjoying life. Such is not the case. Rather, following these principles will ultimately bring you more freedom and the energy to enjoy it.

As you become leaner, more active, dynamic and strong, your future will become even brighter. In any case, these principles are not ultimatums. They do not need to be strictly adhered to 24 hours a day, seven days a week for the rest of your life. Yes, the closer you follow all of them, the better. However, if you can habituate the first six, you will be living on a solid health foundation. All of them are important, but if you can solidify the first six pillars, the rest of the bricks can be put into place one by one as you steadily build a *mansion of mighty good health* that you will live in for the rest of your days. Remember the three little Pigs!

Pillars and Bricks versus Straw and Sticks

1. Put your goal in writing. This principle is well established in the business world as a key to success. We explore this subject at greater length in an upcoming chapter, but to ignore this first step is a mistake. It takes guts, brains and faith to put in writing what you want to achieve. Only a very small percentage of people in the world actually systematically write down their goals, and they leave everyone else in the dust when it comes to performance in their particular field of endeavor. If you have never done this before, you are in for a pleasant surprise. I suggest that your healthiness goal not be entirely appearance focused. For example, do not simply say, "I want to wear a size   pants, etc." That may be a part of your goal, but it is better to include at least one or two performance aspects into your goal(s) as well. For example, "I would like to increase my golf drive by 5 yards and be able to easily complete 25 pushups". This way, you have several ways to measure progress. Page 299 has a form for goal setting.

2. Workout consistently and correctly. If you have read this far, you know what this means by now. This is what separates those who are truly seeking to improve their health, from those who just want to talk about it. Most of the more popular programs, as you know, will not make working out/exercising a condition of their program. That is because they only want your money. Getting fit is a 20/40/40 ratio. First comes the attitude, next the exercise, and last the eating part. Do the hardest stuff first, and the rest is easier. It's kind of like when we were kids. Before you could eat your dessert or go out and play, you had to eat your vegetables.

There have been periods in my life where I have not eaten very well. In fact, I paid little attention to how I ate. When I have done this, I usually put on a few pounds and don't feel as good as normal. But during these times, I continued to workout. I doubt a week has gone by where I have not worked out at least twice. As a result, I continue to maintain or even add to my foundational layer of muscle. Because I maintain the engine of my body (muscle), anytime I want to shed some extra fat I can simply crank up my engine a little through a little more intensive workouts for a week or two. I watch my food intake, and voila, the fat drops off like water off a duck. It's as if you were driving your corvette down the highway. You know you could hit 120 mph by simply pushing a little harder on the accelerator. The resources are in place to increase your performance if desired. On the other hand, simply giving a low performing car a shiny new coat of paint (dieting without exercising), just gives you a mirage of better performance. Mirages are a startling disappointment. Start and stay with exercising correctly and consistently, and you can look forward to an outstanding oasis of well-being.

3. Strength train first, cardio second. This section will be kept super short as you've already heard the good news of what strength training can do for you. It will improve virtually every area of your life (up to 40 benefits), but specifically your strength, stamina, and suppleness. I simply included it here again as a reminder, and for those who may be reading this as an excerpt from my book. One of the reasons that I put this section before the food is that by strength training we will make the cells of the body "hungry" for good nutrition. The cells will be looking for some high quality building blocks to recreate themselves after training. The body will send a message to the brain saying, "feed me, and feed me well!" You can achieve incredible improvements by an effective strength-training program alone. And for many, strength training alone may be enough for the first year or so. But, I would recommend, for those seeking the best that eventually you take up some body weight exercises as well, including calisthenics such as pushups, bodyweight squats, etc. I personally do about 15 minutes of bodyweight exercises on my non-weight training days, and I really enjoy the effect they have. You can find some of my favorites in the workout section of this book.

"Aerobic/cardio" exercise should be included at some point. Never exceed thirty minutes. 12-20 minutes of higher intensity will provide significant benefit for most of us. I always try to do my "cardio" right after strength training, when fat-burning potential is at its highest. For more information on cardio, refer to the workout section of this book.

If you do *nothing* else I recommend in this book though, at least strength train. Every day that goes by that you don't strength train, you are losing muscle. Our society is so automated that most of our muscles have no idea they even exist. You will feel much better and your overall life will be better if you strength train consistently and correctly. Strength train with enthusiasm, intensity, and discipline. Remember, you don't have to exercise . . . you get to!

4. Eat breakfast within 15 minutes of waking up. "What? Are you crazy? I hate, can't, don't and have never eaten breakfast!"' These are the types of comments I hear at nearly every seminar I conduct. Ironically, the ones making such comments often are school food service professionals (my peers) who are in the business of promoting the benefits of eating breakfast! Go figure! But it is clear. Those who are obese and struggling with excess fat problems are often found to have three common factors in their lives. One, they do not exercise habitually. Two, they have no system in place to track their exercise progress or what they eat. And third, they do not eat breakfast. Why eat breakfast so soon after waking up you ask? Because if you do not feed your body soon after getting out of bed, your body goes into "fat storage mode" and your metabolism slows down. If you have trouble thinking of what to eat or the thought of eating that early does not appeal to you, never fear, I have some ideas that can help. But this "eating breakfast immediately" issue is crucial. Like all else worthy in life, you can eventually overcome this problem if you dedicate yourself to making it a habit. We always tell our kids, "eat your breakfast" and then we whine about having to do the same thing.

All the current talk about childhood obesity bothers me. Yes, it is truly a problem that needs attention. But the *REAL* problem is the adults and our attitudes and behavior. Young people *will* follow our lead. Sometimes it takes them a while but eventually most will follow a worthwhile good example. Eat your breakfast. It will make your life better. Eat it a little earlier each day as you work towards the 15 minute goal.

5. Eat 5-8 smaller, equally sized meals per day, every 2-3.5 hours. Follow the wisdom of babies. They instinctively eat every 2.5-3.5 hours. They also eat only enough to satisfy their appetite, energy and growth needs. Breastfeeding babies are perhaps the best example. Their diet naturally includes a high dose of protein, moderate carbs, and an essential amount of healthy fat! We, as adults, however, have screwed up our natural eating patterns and look at most of us. We somehow devised a regimen of skipping breakfast, having a medium sized lunch and a dinner that sometimes goes late into the night. Let's return to our younger years. Ideally, you will want to begin eating an earlier breakfast and then eat again every 2.5-3.5 hours for best results. It is better to eat too soon (2 hours) rather than too late (more than 3.5 hours). If your stomach is growling, then eat a meal, and get back onto the 2.5/3.5 hour track. If you are not hungry after 3.5 hours, have a proper feeding anyway. Your metabolism will slow otherwise. It is important to remember our new definition of a feeding or what we used to call a meal. From now on, a "meal" is defined as anytime you put ANY food in your mouth. The concepts of "lunch" and "dinner" will not hold as much power. Instead, you will begin to think about meal numbers: meal #1, meal #2 . . . . You can still sit down for "lunch" or "dinner" as they correspond with your meal numbers and time frames. But lunch and dinner will be just words and you won't eat any more then than you do at the other meals. If this seems unnatural to you, remember that the current cultural practice of eating large meals late in the day has contributed to the problems with weight and health we have now. Several hundred years ago, when lifestyles were far more physically demanding, larger meals were eaten in the early part of the day.

Some of you may be thinking that this sounds like a hassle, maybe expensive and too much work. Well, dying twenty to thirty years ahead of schedule or enduring the consequences of a chronic disease that severely limits your life for several decades doesn't feel like a great alternative either. And, both of those consequences are real possibilities if we don't pay closer attention to what we put in our bodies. If we don't experience such dire consequences, we are still likely to mire in mediocre health much of the time, at least in comparison to the awesome health available to us. Admittedly though, it does take a little time and work to figure it out at first. But trust me, it will quickly become a habitual lifestyle. Most of us have been incorrectly programmed. I cannot stress enough how important it is to eat smaller meals more frequently. University studies and countless testimonies all indicate that those who do so gain the following benefits:

- **Consume fewer overall calories than those who eat less often. (They don't binge feed)**
- **Shed excess body fat while retaining more muscle.**
- **Maintain proper, safe & healthy blood sugar levels and energy.**
- **Increase their metabolism. Eating /digesting food burns up to 20% of our daily calories!**
- **Have healthier digestion. Smaller meals, more often, continually pushes food through your system. This reduces the possibility of colon cancer and supply's constant nutrients to our cells.**
- **Are more successful in adding muscle. Small, frequent meals (SFM) are known to keep nitrogen levels steady in the bloodstream, which is a key factor to building and maintaining muscle. Eating 5-8 times a day enhances muscle growth up to 30 percent.**

As for the cost, I believe you will find that after you stop buying processed, packaged and prepared foods, you will actually save a little money! But, for the sake of argument, let's say your expenses do go up. I would ask you, what could be more important than what goes into your body? It is understood that most people don't pay close attention to what they eat. But do we really want to be like most people? Most people are unfit, over-fat, overstressed, overtired, and suffering from one or more chronic and perhaps life threatening diseases. This is especially true for most of us over the age of 35. By eating as suggested, you can dramatically improve your health. You can become fit, less fat, less stressed, less tired, and less diseased.

By the way, a few of the other popular fitness and diet books teach the same "smaller, frequent meal" concept as what I'm telling you. But know this: none of us actually invented this method. Instead, it was pioneered in the world of bodybuilding. If you think about it, who would be more interested in reducing excess body fat, building muscle, and having high energy levels and health than a bodybuilder? We can learn from them and vastly improve our lives by utilizing this lifestyle eating technique. I think it is more than worth it and I am quite confident you will soon feel the same way. A little later, I will show you some simple and effective tips for success when it comes to what foods to eat and what meals should look like.

6. Eat *MORE* real, fresh food and less refined, human altered foods. The best general rule is this: Eat like a caveperson. If you can't pick it from a plant, pull it from the ground, milk it from an animal or catch it, don't eat it! Ask yourself, if I were a cave dwelling person, or simply lost in the mountains, what would I eat? Chances are it

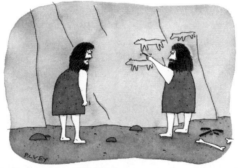

"My doctor says you should be drawing more fruits and vegetables."

would not be in a bag or fortified to taste sweet! Anthropologists suggest that early human's diets consisted mainly of meat, nuts/seeds, vegetables and fruits. And, there weren't any pictures of out-of-shape, obese people on the walls of caves were there?

This eating like an early human idea has actually resulted in a diet called the "Caveman Diet". Some refer to it as the Paleolithic Diet and there are several books outlining its concepts. One of the books is titled, *Neanderthin*. The general theory of eating "natural" foods makes sense, but it also seems that some of these "Paleo only" practioners go a little too far in deciding which foods the early humans consumed. Truly, who can know for sure which plants or animals early humans ate? The strict "caveman" diet, for instance, eliminates all dairy and wheat products. According to the devout cave eating advocates, these products did not exist in an edible form in pre-historic times. It seems like these folks may be going a little too far. Eat real foods, in as close as possible to their natural state. By the time we get to most of our food, it has been so re-defined, processed, and altered from its original state that it is doubtful our body recognizes it as food! Often these are foods that come in a bag, wrapper, box, package or can. Foods altered and stripped by humans are less beneficial to our bodies. The proof is in the pudding. Nearly every health and physical ailment we currently suffer from in this country is related to the food we eat and our lack of exercise. Bottom line: eat **REAL** foods. This includes the following:

A) **Lean proteins:** (4-6 portions daily), 2-6 oz depending on your size. I can hear the screams now. We often hear that we get all the protein we need from a "normal" diet. The question is, what is normal? Do we want to be normal? Our goal is to take our health to the highest-level possible, to regenerate our bodies and restore lean tissue. My experience has been that most people don't eat enough lean protein, especially many women. Protein fuels metabolism, requires more calories to digest, stimulates the release of glucagon (a fat burning hormone), builds lean tissue (muscle and bone), repairs and builds the *entire* body, including hormones, the brain, and the immune system. Those who do not eat enough protein are hurting their health . . . period. How much is enough? I recommend that those who strength train eat a ½—1 gram of protein per pound of their **lean bodyweight goal.** For example, my lean bodyweight goal is 180 pounds. Thus, I generally eat 90 to 180 grams of protein per day, and have for twenty plus years. So far, the kidneys and liver and everything else are just fine.

Include turkey, chicken, lean beef, tuna, lean pork, eggs, ham (low/no sugar), cottage cheese, all sea food (not fried), whey protein, skim milk. Vegetarians should at least eat eggs, soy, and cottage cheese.

B) **Fibrous carbohydrates:** (6-10 portions daily). **Primarily from fresh or frozen whole vegetables and fruits.** Focus on vegetables (too many to list). I suggest 3 portions of veggies to each fruit. The reason for this suggestion is that most of us do the opposite. With fruit, work on more berries (blue, straw, black and rasp) with no sugar added. They are high in fiber and other awesome phyto-chemicals. You cannot eat too much green, leafy, high fiber vegetables. My personal favorite is fresh spinach. I try to have some with at least three meals daily. Popeye was right.

C) **Starchy carbohydrates:** (1-3 day; 2-4 oz portions). Include whole grain brown rice, oatmeal, baked or boiled skin on potatoes, peas and corn, beans of all types, 100 % whole grain breads and cereals. I know, I know. The pyramid says 6-11. Try 1-2 a day. Get more carbs from veggies. I doubt anyone will dry up and blow away. You will be fine, perhaps even finer.

D) **Fat:** (4-6 day; 1 oz portions). Yes . . . fat! Fat has been considered taboo for decades. This is a mistake. Fat does not make us fat. Too little muscle, inactivity and over indulgence equals obesity and health problems. Include a little natural fat with approximately 4 of your daily 5-8 meals. Fat helps with hormone regulation, nerve transmission and vitamin absorption. It also adds flavor and prevents hunger and food binges. Portions should be about a tablespoon or one ounce per meal. Include real butter, hard and crumbled cheeses, heavy whipping cream, bacon, genuine mayonnaise, sour cream, omega and olive oils, no sugar-added salad dressings, guacamole, olives. With your new, more active muscle building lifestyle, your body can handle this little bit of essential fat.

7. Keep records of food intake and workouts. I have included sheets to track your workouts and eating patterns. This is a key to being successful, especially in regards to food intakes. In fact, this is part of the "big three" in regards to succeeding at becoming lean. The other two are consistent exercise and eating breakfast. You will not need to do this the rest of your life, although it is not a bad idea. I currently don't journal what I eat, but I do keep "notes" of it on my daily planner. I simply jot down what I had to eat and what time. That way I stay on track. It probably takes me less than a minute per day to do this. I always write down my workout results however, as this is my feedback to show progress and stay inspired.

8. Eliminate forever the words "dieting, diet and/or losing weight" from your vocabulary forever. Replace them with, "improved nutritional lifestyle" and "transforming my body composition by restoring lost muscle and reducing excess body fat". Think I'm kidding? To "diet" alone or simply lose weight to become smaller are both foolish and unhealthy behaviors. Quite frankly, dieting alone is for dummies. I know that you and I are not dummies. America, however, is obsessed with becoming smaller. If you have heard me speak, you now know that simply becoming smaller for appearance sake will backfire on you.

9. Establish in your mind more positive and productive healthiness behaviors. Always focus on *actually* improving the health, fitness and functioning of your body first, appearance second. In this day of excessive stomach stapling and plastic surgery's, this concept may be foreign. Nevertheless, it is what will deliver the long term vitality, aliveness and improved appearance we all ultimately want.

10. Junk food night. Enjoy a 1-4 hour period each week to indulge a little. This is a method that I derived from my mothers system of feeding our family a consistently healthy diet while allowing for the occasional splurge. I grew up in a family of seven children, and my mother worked hard to provide us with excellent, nourishing and nutritious foods. But on Saturday evenings, she would break out the chips and dip, sodas, pies, etc. Without trying, we learned to be disciplined with food choices during the week knowing that we could enjoy a treat each weekend with no harm done. I have continued to employ this strategy in my own life, and find it works very well. I recommend you do the same. I am aware that other popular fitness books suggest a similar concept, but I believe that my mother was the originator of the model (just kidding). You too can break all of the food rules one night a week. Try to keep the night consistent and the portions within reason. Have your donuts and pizza. Just don't let it get the worst of you. By the way, "**junk food night**" is just a phrase I coined to signify no restrictions that evening. It does not mean that I consider every thing I eat that evening as "junk". In fact, there is a particular donut my family and I periodically enjoy called a Super Donut. It is a favorite in our house and is fortified with protein, vitamins and minerals while being hearty and *very* good.

The purpose of this night is to help you be disciplined the rest of the week and to enjoy your favorite treats once a week. You can enjoy them knowing that your new and improved fat-incinerating metabolism can handle these foods during this pre-planned period of indulgence!

11. Igloo coolers are a body's best friend. Plan your meals out. Invest in a small igloo cooler and some Tupper ware that you can take to work and in your car. Do not settle for low quality nutrition. The few minutes needed to prepare ahead of time is worth it. My cooler is always stocked with a few foods that require no heating or additional preparation.

12. Reduce or eliminate all starchy carbohydrates the last one or two meals before bedtime to shed fat quicker and keep it off. There is no need to go to the extreme of no or tremendously low-carb plans. This will be explored in more detail throughout this section of the book, but suffice it to say that we can stay quite lean by simply eating carbs during the earlier hours of the day (before 3-5:00 pm). I suggest you still include high fiber green vegetables for dinner and evening snacks. You will see examples of this in the seven-day feeding outline.

13. Determine your approximate calorie target per day. To do this, first determine your "ideal lean body weight goal" (ILBWG). This is the only time we will discuss body weight as our real interest is BODY COMPOSITION. For now though, we need a measuring stick. So, choose a realistic body weight goal which you feel would be ideal for you (lean, healthy, energetic and a good appearance). For example, mine is 180 lbs. Now, take that number, and simply place a "0" after it. For me, that number would be 1800. That is the base amount of calories my body needs each day to maintain 180 pounds of lean, healthy bodyweight. I suggest you give yourself about a 300 calorie "buffer". So, in my case, I would eat approximately 1800-2100 calories per day.

Your numbers will most likely be different. A few cautions though. Do not get too hung up or obsessed with numbers. It is suggested that you monitor your calories per meal for the first 4-6 weeks until you have a good feel for how large your meals should be. After that, you will instinctively know how much to have per "feeding". When introducing new foods into your menu, however, you will still want to read the label to monitor the calories. Many of you will want to know the breakdown of protein, fat, and carbohydrates suggested. As such, I have included the following page for you to plug your own "numbers" into. Later in this section of the book, I address the percentages for protein, fat, and carbohydrates recommended in more detail. Even if you don't like the percentages suggested, do the calculations following the formula below for now. You can adjust it later on if you desire.

Approximate calories per day/meal Formula

1. Your ideal lean body goal: _____   Fred's ideal lean body weight: 180

2. Establish your calories per day minimum by tacking   Fred's calories per day: 1800-2100
    on a "0" to your Goal, Plus a 300 Cal "Buffer". Do not
    go below your minimum!   Your calories per day: _____

3. Establish your calories per meal by dividing total   *1800 calories , 6 meals = 300 calories per "meal" or feeding*
    calories per day by the number of meals you will have
    (i.e.: 6-8):   _____ calories , 6 meals =
          _____   _____ calories per meal

4. Establish your daily protein requirement by simply   *Fred's ideal lean body weight = 180 lbs.*
    entering your ideal body weight again: *Daily protein needs = 180 grams*
          _____   *Total grams , 6 meals = 30 grams*

                                              Your ideal lean body weight = _____ lbs.
                                              Daily protein needs = grams per meal
                                              Total grams _____ , # ____ meals = _____
                                                           grams protein per meal

5. Establish your daily fat requirement by multiplying   *1800 calories x .03 = 54 grams fat per day*
    .03 by your total daily calories. This gives you your   *54 , 4 meals with fat = 14 grams per meal*
    daily fat gram goal. Divide that number by the number
    of meals to see how many fat grams to have per meal.   _____ daily calories x .03 = _____ grams fat per day
                                              _____ , # ____ meals = _____ grams fat per meal

6. Establish your daily carb requirement by multiplying   *1800 calories x .0825 = 148 grams carb per day*
    .0825 by your total daily calories goal. Divide the   *148 , 4 meals = 37 grams per meal*
    answer by the number of meals to see how many carb
    grams to have with each carb meal.   _____ calories x .0825 = _____ grams carb per day
                                              _____ , # _____ meals = _____ grams carb per meal

*Remember, women should never go below **1300 K per day**, and men not below **1500 K per day**, no matter your size or goal. **The numbers above are simply guidelines**. The most important thing is to **focus** on the **first six pillars** of the 21 Principles !*

14. Determine your approximate calorie target per meal. This is easy. Now that you know your approximate calories (K) per day (from above), you simply divide that by six (or 7 to 8 depending on how often you want to eat) and that is your calorie target per meal. You will be surprised how quickly your body adapts to, enjoys and thrives with this method.

15. Watch for "brain suckers" and other hidden dangers. One thing myself and other health/fitness researchers feel is contributing to our current poor health plague is the hidden ingredients that are put into nearly every processed/packaged food you can buy. Many of these ingredients were unheard of 30 years ago. They include: high fructose corn syrup, corn syrup, corn syrup solids, hydrogenated and partially hydrogenated oils/fats, etc. These ingredients are subtle "dangers" that do not contribute to becoming lean and healthy. They should be eliminated or at least significantly reduced from your food intake. And according to Dr. Diana Schwarzbein (Scwarzbein Factor), some of these ingredients contribute to poor health and accelerated aging by stimulating an insulin response which in turn stimulates a secretion of serotonin from the brain, which creates a vicious cycle of insulin response, serotonin stimulation, brief energy high, depleted energy, lethargy, depression or stress, turning to stimulants, elevated insulin, etc. Thus, I have dubbed these ingredients, along with added refined sugars of any type and the stimulants of caffeine, alcohol and nicotine as "brain suckers'. Imagine energy and life, for that matter, being slowly sucked out of your brain every time you artificially stimulate insulin or stress response through ingestion of these questionable ingredients. In reality, when we voluntarily submit ourselves to these substances, we may be actually slowly and prematurely sucking the life out of ourselves. I know that sounds somewhat harsh, but I feel it is a good and accurate description and picture of what many of us do to ourselves, sometimes daily.

Even artificial sweeteners are able to contribute to insulin response, according to Schwarzbein. Admittedly, this didn't make sense to me, as these artificial sweeteners are not actually sugar. Dr. Schwarzbein explains how the brain/body cannot differentiate between where the "sweet" flavor comes from, and thus reacts with an elevation of insulin response. As I pondered this thesis, I thought of at least three people I know who have confessed to being "addicted" to diet sodas. One gentleman told me that he cannot make it through his day without his 12 pack of diet soda, while another woman refers often to her "diet soda Jones" (meaning her fix). So, either the soda manufactures are placing an addictive substance in the diet sodas, or this craving for these products is tied to the artificial sweetener, which in turn creates this insulin response, etc. The insulin response theory seems more likely. Either way, a continual diet of artificial sweeteners *cannot* benefit the body, and we would all be wise to at least reduce if not totally eliminate their use.

Thus, the recommendation is to cut back on stimulants, added sugars and artificial fats and sweeteners as much as possible. Many of us may need to progressively do this, versus trying to go "cold turkey". Coffee is one of my personal struggles, and my goal is to keep consumption at two cups per day or less. Alcohol has no true redeeming value, except to provide a temporary escape. Just be careful how far and how often you escape! In regards to smoking, I am aware that this is an extremely difficult habit to quit. But one does have to ask the person who smokes, "do you really not like yourself that much?" Smoking, or cigarettes has been accurately described as coffin nails, cancer sticks and long barreled suicide. It is simply a matter of time before you will get "nailed" by the cigarettes. Start strength training and exercising today, and your body will *beg* you to quit and start feeding it some healthy food and oxygen instead.

16. Supplements. Most supplements are unnecessary. You can get all you need from a good fitness program and eating effectively. No supplement can really make up for a substandard lifestyle. The people selling them won't tell us that of course, but it is a fact. Follow the exercise program in this book, along with the feeding formula. Then take a high quality vitamin-mineral pill and perhaps some essential fatty acid oil if your diet is low in fish and you should be good to go. I do use and recommend whey protein powder, but that is actually a high quality, natural convenience "food", not a supplement.

17. Focus on portions, not servings. For example, we are often told that we need to eat a half-cup of this or a half-cup of that. Personally, I don't always want to eat a half-cup of broccoli with a meal, for example. So, I will eat 4-5 florets instead. Many people I have worked with avoid vegetables like the plague. Part of the reason was that they felt they needed to eat a plateful. When I introduced the concept of just having a little to start with, they began to include more veggies in their daily eating, which is the goal!

18. Learn the food basics of protein, fat & carbohydrates. This is so important, that it should be taught every year k-12. Most of us start to decay before age 30 from poor nutritional habits, so what good does all that reading and writing do us if we can't even read or understand a nutrition label? And that is where I suggest you start. For the next two months, read every label of everything you buy or eat. Concentrate on how much protein, carbohydrates and fat different foods have. Learn how to read labels and understand percentages. E-mail me if you need some help (fitfooddude@aol.com). Eight out of ten premature deaths and disabling diseases in this country are directly related to poor nutrition and inactivity. People tend to worry more about the type of gas they put in their car than what they put into their bodies. Rather than spend thirty minutes on mindless television, let's take a few minutes to learn the basics of protein, fats, and carbohydrates. It will improve current functioning and could extend our lives by 15-20 years or more!

19. Measure what you can. Being neurotic is not encouraged, but it is important to measure as much of your food as possible, especially at the beginning. The degree to which this must be done varies from person to person. Some folks really struggle with getting lean, and thus having a more precise measurement of amounts of food is needed to help them succeed. In time, you will get a good feel for amounts, but be diligent at first. In some cases with people failing to make progress, a key contributor has been found to be over and underestimating amounts of food eaten. Details can make the difference.

20. Fill up on fiber. Fiber comes primarily from fresh/frozen vegetables, fruits, beans, and *true* whole grains. It helps us function properly and assists our health dramatically. Shoot for at least thirty grams per day. A good fiber supplement can be helpful here. Try to use one that is as natural as possible, but do not overuse these. Still, the goal is real food. I use a product called "Benefiber" with my whey protein drinks. Slowly work your way towards 70 grams per day.

21. Find a partner, coach, or at least an encourager. Seek out a positive person who is disciplined and determined to get the most out of life. Someone who is "walking the wellness talk", works out, will be honest with you, and wants the *best* for you. Ask them to either help you, train with you, or at least keep you accountable. If you need more ideas of how to meet this need, you can e-mail me at *fitfooddude@aol.com.*

Chapter 18

To Be Terrific, You Must Be Specific

Now that we have looked at the "Fit Food Dude Formula" to becoming a "LFIAAWM" in a little more detail, it is time to put it into practice. We will do this by first building a shopping list of staple foods that you will want to have in your home and eat the majority of time. After we go through these shopping lists, we will review a weekly menu so that you can get an idea of what successful eating looks like. This seems to be most helpful to the most people, as it gives them a pattern to follow. By now, you should have a pretty good idea of what is expected. There is no way that what I have written into my weekly menu will appeal to everyone's appetite or favorite foods. Having been in the food business for nearly thirty years, I am all too aware of how difficult it is to please everyone with food choices. Therefore, you can make adjustments to these foods if you wish. Simply make sure that the foods you select are similar in their nutritional profile.

As of this writing, I have not included specific recipes. There are many recipe books available, many geared toward healthier, lower fat and lower carb dishes. Some of those books can offer suggestions or dishes that you can incorporate into my formula. As you will see, however, most of my "meals" are not what we have been programmed to think of as meals. The majority of the food I eat requires no heating, cooking or actual preparation. Dinner is the main food event in our home, and we usually prepare enough to provide at least a few more meals the next couple of days. Thus, there is not a great need for countless recipes. Besides, most of the people I know don't seem to have the time to prepare extensive recipes anyway. Having said all that, as I come across and develop my own recipes, I will post them on my website and include them in future editions of this book. From this day forward though, it is strongly suggested that you spend most of your food money and digestive activity with the following friends of your body.

Lean Proteins 4-6 Servings/"Portions" Per day

- Skinless Chicken (Not fried, includes both white and dark meat)
- Skinless Turkey (white/dark meat)
- Whey protein powder This is a real food. It is a pure, natural, high quality protein isolated from cow's milk. It is also a complete protein, containing the 8 essential amino acids. There are however, various types and qualities on the market. To learn more, visit *www.wheyoflife.org*.
- Lean Beef (top sirloin, ground beef, flank steak, etc)
- Eggs (three whites to one yolk)
- Tuna packed in water
- Lean trimmed Pork roast/chops
- All fish and seafood (not breaded/deep fried)
- Salmon, Sardines
- Non/low fat cottage cheese
- Cream cheese, non-fat
- Skim milk
- Tofu
- Soy Protein
- Lean Ham (low sugar)
- Lamb
- Ground turkey
- Turkey burgers
- Jerky (low fat and sugar)

Vegetables (high fiber/low sugar carbs) At *least* 3-6 times per day, can be unlimited!

- Fresh Spinach
- Broccoli
- Bell Peppers
- Celery
- Onion
- Mushrooms
- Asparagus
- Zucchini
- Green beans
- Cucumber
- Cauliflower
- Sprouts
- Watercress
- Cabbage
- Peppers of all kinds (jalapeno, habanera, cayenne)
- All leafy greens

Fresh Fruit (& a few other higher sugar, simple but natural, clean (minimal human altering carbs) (2 portions per day)

- Apples
- Oranges
- Blueberries
- Strawberries
- Any Berries! (unsweetened)
- Bananas
- Pears
- Cantaloupe/honeyde w/watermelon
- All unsweetened fruits
- Non-fat yogurt (Mixed with fruit)
- Natural Pure Honey or *Pure* Maple Syrup (a teaspoon or so mixed with fruit is o.k.)
- Tomatoes
- Carrots (higher in natural sugars)
- Skim milk

Starchy, complex carbs (1-3 portions per day)

- Whole grain brown rice
- Odwalla Bar (Cherry C Monster is my favorite)—Found in health food section.
- Fiber One cereal
- Old fashioned or razor cut oats
- 100 % Whole grain bagel
- Shredded wheat and bran cereal (This is an actual product w/ no added sugar)

- Cereals that contain no added sugar, fructose etc, and that are 100% whole grain
- Natural unbuttered plain popcorn
- Corn or peas
- Beans of all types (no sugar or fat added, instead use seasonings & spices, including salsa). Small red beans are especially high in fiber.
- Baked or boiled potatoes with skin on.
- Yams/sweet potato
- Pastas, preferably whole grain or vegetable based.
- 100 % whole grain, natural breads (the less commercial, the better. Commercial bread products often contain high fructose corn syrup and preservatives).

Fats (4 "portions" per day) Keep portions of fat under control. I recommend not more than one ounce or one tablespoon of fat per feeding, and at a ratio of one fat gram to every three grams of protein per meal. If you are not a numbers person, always try to have three times as many protein calories as fat calories. For example, the portion of protein on your plate (chicken breast) should be at least three times as big as the fat portion on your plate (salad dressing). This is just to give you a concept to follow; obviously it will not always be a hard and fast rule. Also, it is a good idea to get 2/3 of your fat from unsaturated sources, and about 1/3 from saturated sources. For the most part, fat from animals is saturated, and non-animal sources are unsaturated.

Unsaturated Fats

- Essential fatty acid oil (Omega 3 fatty acids, omega 6 fatty acids, omega 9 fatty acids)
- Avocado
- Real mayonnaise
- Olives
- Virgin Olive oil
- Salad dressings: ranch, Caesar, blue cheese, etc. I try to use as natural as possible, with minimal ingredients and no added sweeteners. Limit to one-two tablespoons and best if kept on the side for dipping.

Saturated Fats

- Cream cheese
- Heavy whipping cream
- Crumbled blue cheese
- Real butter
- Any hard cheese
- Sour cream
- Bacon

Nuts, Nut Butters, & Seeds (*Once per day*) Nuts, seeds or nut butters are kind of an oddball food. It is suggested that they are eaten alone, as a meal. Once per day at most, however, and don't go crazy on them. These foods are high in fat and calories so remember you're "per feeding" calorie guidelines.

- Dry roasted & lightly salted almonds (almonds are the most nutrient dense and highest fiber nut).
- Natural Peanut Butter (I prefer smooth organic, as long as its unsweetened and no hydrogenated oils added). Many clients really like just having 2-3 tablespoons of straight peanut butter as a meal.
- Sunflower seeds
- Raw Spanish peanuts
- Soy nuts, walnuts, pecans, etc.

Condiments. (unlimited) Avoid condiments that are high in calories, especially from sugars and fat.

- Stone ground mustard
- Unsweetened pickle relish (Bubbies brand is great)
- Unsweetened pickles
- Salsa (unsweetened)

Percentages & Ratios

These days, many people seem to want to know the ratios of any nutrition system. This is probably due to the "Zone Diet". It is a *good* idea to know the ratios of protein, carbohydrates, and fat we want to shoot for in our daily eating. One of the mantra's often heard in the world of nutrition is that "calories are calories, you simply need to reduce calories and increase activity in order to become lean and healthy". This statement is only partially true and an overgeneralization. The fact is that each of the macronutrients (Protein, fat, and carbs) has a different impact and are processed and utilized differently by the body. Hence, the Fit Food Formula consists of eating *approximately* **40% protein, 33% carbohydrates, and 27% of calories from fat.** A few people have criticized this formula, saying that it is too high in protein. My responses to these objections are as follows.

1) First off, these are simply guidelines. You can still be successful if you do not follow them, but adhere to the rest of the formula outlined. Some people want to know numbers, so these are what I recommend. All of the "high protein warnings" of what might happen long term, have been heard. Some of these warnings include effect on kidneys, leaching of calcium from bones, etc. All of the warnings include "might happen" statements. Well, as previously mentioned, I have followed these guidelines for almost twenty years. So far, everything is working quite well. If it did not, I would not follow it. Always remember, this formula is a lifestyle that builds muscle (lean tissue), the heart (a muscle!) bones, joints, nerves, ligaments, additional arteries and capillaries. This lifestyle works best with a bit more protein and yes, perhaps the average "normal" person who sits on their duff most of the time could get by with less. This is not a "less" lifestyle. It is a lifestyle of *more* life, energy, and vitality. If this feels like too much protein, however, simply eat a little less protein and a little more of the foods from each of the other categories and continue to workout consistently, effectively and with some passion. I *do not* eat 40% of my calories each and every day from protein, although it is a goal. Some days I eat less, some day's maybe a little more.

As a side note, one of my most successful students never ate more than 25 % of her calories from protein. However, when I met her she was probably consuming less than 10 % of her calories from protein. To make matters worse, she was skipping breakfast and only eating twice a day, lunch and dinner. In addition, the only exercising she was doing was using a treadmill. She was a stubborn individual, but I was able to convince her to at least *double* her current protein intake, start eating breakfast, double her meals to four times per day and to lift weights three days per week. In a little over six months she lost 55 pounds of excess body fat and *added* 15 pounds of life giving and preserving muscle.

The point is this. Some of you may object to the higher protein suggestions. The tale of this woman has been told to illustrate that even if you don't follow the exact guidelines, you can still be successful. Perhaps you will *NEVER* eat 40% of your calories from protein. I only recommend it to those who want to know what I think is *best* for getting as lean, fit and strong as they possibly can. I am open to a person eating less than 40% of calories from protein, but an effective form of strength training, having smaller meals more often, and eating a high quality breakfast are essential and not usually open to negotiation. Protein amounts, however, are an area where modifications can be made.

2) *Most* who criticize higher protein amounts know little, if anything, about strength training or how to build muscle (lean tissue). Because we now know how crucial muscle (lean tissue!) is to our health and fitness, a person who does not have relevant experience in the relationship of protein, strength training and muscle (lean tissue) building is not in a position to help us much. You will often hear "experts" saying that those who desire to build extra muscle or strength do not require any additional protein in their diet. However, in my experience, rarely has this person actually added any additional muscle or strength to his or her own body!

3) Millions of Americans are buying into the NO or LOW carb, high protein AND high fat Atkins diet and simply becoming smaller, fatter, weaker and unhealthier people. My approach is balanced and sensible, incorporating higher protein, lower refined carbs, and moderate natural fat. Bottom line is that it will make you leaner, stronger, fitter and healthier, not like Atkins or any other diet-only scheme.

4) Ask any critics to show you one legitimate peer reviewed research article *proving* **that up to 40% of calories from protein is harmful to your health in the short or long term.** Many critics of higher protein intakes cite "potential" long-term damage to kidneys, bones, etc. Hundreds of thousands of athletes have been eating higher amounts of protein than the RDA for decades, yet not one healthy, trained individual has ever suffered a kidney failure or liver problem associated with too high of protein intake. I am not, however, suggesting that everyone indiscriminately and without any thought ingest tons of protein into his or her body. No, I suggest you follow this *entire* lifestyle, and eat according to the formulas I've given in combination with your goals, size, activity levels, etc. A respectable amount of lean protein is the *least* of most people's health concerns.

5) What do critics look like in a swimsuit? I know this is not supposed to be about appearance, but wouldn't you agree that it gets a little old listening to supposed nutrition and health experts who look like they couldn't punch their way out of a paper bag or do 10 pushups to save their life? So yes, we must do a quick analysis of the expert's condition. Are they lean, strong, fit and healthy? Do they look pretty darn good for their age? Can they do things physically most people their age cannot? If so, perhaps give them your ear for a while. If not, let's proceed. Something must change. Couches are coming and bringing more diabetes, more cancer, and more lethargy. More boxed cereals and bagged breads is not the answer.

A question I often get is, "what do you eat each day?" I am going to share with you what the "formula" I have used and taught others looks like in real life. It has been my experience that by simply outlining what to eat each day, others are able to get the idea, and be successful. As you read this, remember that I weigh about 180/ 185 pounds. Modify your intake based upon your personal goals. The following is what I call, "The Fit Food Feeding Formula" ™ and with it you can enjoy a superior degree of healthiness for the rest of your life.

One Week example of the "*Fit Food Feeding Formula*"
Water throughout the day between meals. I generally drink at
least two quarts per day, even up to and before bedtime.

Day one *Monday*

4:30 am	Glass of water and Lean Body Latte' (see page 189)
6:00-6:25	**Strength training/weight lifting**
6:25-6:40	**Jog, sprints, or recumbent bike**
7:00 am	Non fat plain yogurt, 6-7 fresh strawberries, a teaspoon of pure maple syrup and a small glass of water with 2 vitamin pills.
9:30 am	¾ cup of dry roasted almonds (sometimes salted too)
12:30 pm	Leftover Broiled beef patty, fresh spinach, broccoli, bell peppers, and a tablespoon of ranch dressing
3:30 pm	Nonfat cottage cheese and ½ apple
6:30 pm	Grilled mahi-mahi, green beans, fresh carrots, spinach, essential fatty acid oil (tablespoon), blue cheese crumbles (1/2-1 ounce), 2 vitamin pills

Day two *Tuesday*

5:00 am	Water and Cup of coffee
5:15 am	Two tablespoons of natural organic creamy peanut butter and skim milk
6:45-7:00 am	**Body weight exercises, including chair pushups, deep knee bends, and bridging.** Your regimen may be different, depending upon your fitness levels.
7:30 am	Old fashioned Oatmeal (1/2 cup dry), heated in water, small handful fresh/frozen blueberries, teaspoon of pure maple syrup, 2 vitamin pills
10:30 am	Chocolate Mocha Whey Protein (46 grams of protein or 2 scoops), mixed with ice water, heavy whipping cream, and *Benefiber*

1:30 pm	Roasted Turkey in light sugar free gravy with a salad of fresh spinach, broccoli, celery and a few jalapeño peppers sprinkled with grated cheddar and a tablespoon of ranch dressing. 2 vitamin pills
4:00 pm	Corn and black bean salad with fresh lemon juice, onions, cilantro
6:45 pm	BBQ Skinless chicken thighs, seasoned with Lawry's. Served with Steamed broccoli, a teaspoon of real butter, and a few carrot-eenies. 2 vitamin pills

Day three *Wednesday*

4:30 am	Water & Lean Body Latte
6:00-6:40 am	**Strength training and aerobic exercise**
7:30 am	Whole-wheat bagel, non fat cream cheese, no added sugar raspberry jam, 2 vitamin pills.
10:30 am	A handful of dry roasted almonds (3/4 cup) Remember, I weigh about 185-190 pounds, modify the amount based on your lean bodyweight goal!
1:30 pm	Chicken Chow Mein with just the vegetables. Salad of fresh spinach, broccoli, etc with a little (a tablespoon) ranch dressing on the side
4:00 pm	One small whole apple, skim milk
6:30 pm	Top sirloin steak, broiled, served with green beans, butter, mushrooms, red onion and cilantro. 2 vitamin pills

Day Four *Thursday*

5:00 am	Water & Cup of coffee
5:15 am	One whole orange, half of a whole grain bagel
6:45-7:00 am	**Bodyweight exercises**
8:15 am	A handful of raw Spanish peanuts and walnuts
10:45 am	Non fat cottage cheese (one cup) with a

	tablespoon of essential fatty acid, sprinkled with cinnamon powder and a few bell pepper strips.
1:45 pm	Steak "Fajita" salad (leftover top sirloin from previous night), bell peppers, onions, mushrooms, tomato, etc and a tablespoon of creamy Caesar dressing.
4:45 pm	Odwalla Fruit bar (Cherry C Monster is my favorite) skim milk
7:45 pm	Omelet (three whites to one yolk, or try eggbeaters) with fresh spinach, green onions, a little Swiss cheese, 2 vitamin pills.

Day Five *Friday*

4:45 am	Water & Lean Body Latte (46 grams high quality protein, 9 grams of fat and 5 grams of carbs)
6:00-6:40 am	**Strength train and cardio/aerobic**
7:15 am	Fiber one cereal, skim milk, unsweetened raspberries, raisins, 2 vitamin pills.
10:15 am	Dry roasted, salted almonds
1:15 pm	Tuna salad with tomato, celery, stone ground mustard, real mayo, unsweetened pickle, cilantro and two vitamin pills
4:00 pm	One whole fresh pear, cottage cheese, a half of an orange.
6:30 pm	Pepperoni Pizza, French fries, diet coke, chocolate chip cookie.

Remember, this is my "junk food night (JFN)". I allow myself this indulgence period from 5:00 pm Friday till about 9:00 pm Friday. Other favorite indulgence meals include "full on" Mexican or Italian dinners, hamburgers and fries, an occasional beer, and of course, ice cream. Some have suggested to me that this is not a good idea, as these foods are "bad for your health", or that for people with eating disorders, this practice could cause problems. It is simply a method that has worked for many people. It has worked for me. There are certain foods I like occasionally, that if I ate consistently, would mess up my health. Once a week, I can track and maintain on a reasonable level. If you overdo it on this night, you will probably feel like crud the next day, and next time you will be smart enough to be more controlled. One thing is for sure. This JFN practice sure beats feeling guilty about "blowing it" in the middle of the week. By setting up a time when you know you can "party" a little, the pressure is off. If a person has an eating disorder, this might not be for them. But, it could me modified to fit into their approach for improvement.

Day Six *Saturday*

6:00 am	Coffee
6:15 am	Peanut Butter
7:45-8:00 am	**Body weight exercises**
8:45 am	Pancakes, Pure Maple syrup, bananas, fresh strawberries
11:45 am	Skim milk (8 grams serving) with banana whey protein powder and 2 vitamin pills
2:00 pm	Ground Turkey & lean beef lasagna made with spinach noodles, vegetables, low fat mozzarella, ricotta and cottage cheese.
4:45 pm	Deviled eggs, low fat turkey salami, sugarless pickle slices
7:00 pm	BBQ Chicken breast, asparagus spears with butter, 2 vitamin pills

Day Seven Sunday

6:00 am	Water & Lean Body Latte
No exercise, a day of rest. I will do something "physical ?" like fishing or boating with the family and friends after church.	
8:30 am	No added sugar cereal, skim milk, fresh strawberries, and banana
12:00 pm	Lean ground turkey on a baked potato, with broccoli, mushrooms, green onions, salsa and a little (teaspoon) real sour cream. 2 vitamin pills
3:00 pm	Whole apple, plain yogurt

6:00 pm	Fresh broiled salmon with zucchini, bell pepper, onions, cilantro sautéed in virgin olive oil. 2 vitamin pills.
8:30 pm	Two Tablespoons Peanut butter and celery sticks

Hopefully this gives you the idea. Obviously, you may not like the foods I do. Thus, you may have to make substitutions. This lifestyle soon becomes a habit that will serve you mighty good health for decades to come. There are no complicated regimes or counting needed once you understand the basic guidelines. Simply follow the formulas given you up to this point. Let's summarize them one more time in order to reinforce them, as well as offer insights on frequently asked questions and popular topics of nutrition that many people have inquired about.

Take Home Points

- Drink water & eat something decent as soon as possible (absolutely no later than 30 minutes) upon arising. (See my examples)
- Exercise at least three days per week, every other day and that needs to include strength building. Do not miss workouts for lame reasons. We are talking about your life here.
- Eat smaller, equally sized "meals/feedings" every 2.5-3.5 hours
- Eat more real food.
- If you want to reduce carbs, try reducing fake refined ones. Atkins and similar concepts have gone *too* far in carb reduction, especially concerning whole natural fruit. Carbs were created for a reason, and are needed by the body. Apples were not made to rot on trees, etc. It is a good idea to get *more* of your carbs from fresh, high fiber green leafy vegetables, fresh whole fruits (not juices sold by blender people), and things you can pick or pull and then eat in their natural state with minimal preparation. This includes fresh corn, beans, etc. And on occasion, 100 % whole grain breads, whole grain brown rice, baked skin-on potatoes, etc.

- "Sandwich" your nutrients. What this means is to try and make your first and last meals of the day primarily from proteins with a little fat. Why? Because doing so helps jump-start the metabolism first thing in the morning and protein is needed during sleep to help grow, maintain and repair the body. Carbohydrates main function is that of energy. Thus, I recommend consuming the majority of your carbohydrates in the mid morning and early afternoon. Try not to eat complex, starchy carbs after 5:00 pm and you will be far finer and fitter than all of the carb depleted non-exercising smaller fatter people out there. A nutrition educator recently told me that this recommendation did not make "biochemical" sense. We could argue that point, but the point is that this method *works* in helping keep us lean, fit and strong. This same person suggested eating carbohydrates before bedtime to help "calm the nerves" before going to sleep. I told her that I did not eat for stress therapy, but to be fit and healthy. If I feel a need to calm my nerves before going to sleep that means something is wrong in my life, and I should probably figure it out so that I can go to sleep in peace. Elevating ones insulin levels by consuming carbohydrates before they go to bed is not a way to improve ones body composition or health.

- If you *insist* on going very low carb, try instead going lower starchy carbs. That is, reduce breads, potatoes, rice, beans, corn, etc. You should, however, eat lots of high fiber veggies and still eat *whole* fruits. Keep your lean proteins in a 3 to 1 ratio with natural fats and be sure to get 2/3 of your fats from unsaturated natural sources. You will cut the body-fat but preserve your muscle/lean tissue, as well as health and energy levels. This "drop the starches" is a method that I learned in college from my wrestling buddies who had to cut weight while remaining strong and healthy in order to compete. Many have found this a great way to achieve leanness and keep their health and vitality intact. I would say it accurately describes how I eat much of the time, although I have not cut out starchy foods *completely.* I still enjoy high starch complex carbs, usually once-twice per day, but most of the time before 3:00 pm.

- Know approximately how many calories you require per day and per feeding, to build /maintain muscle and keep body fat at low levels.

- Set aside a 1-4 hour time period each week to indulge some in your favorite food that might create problems for you if you ate it all week. Keep the day consistent with an occasional "flex" for your nephews wedding, etc.

- Drink plenty of water. Even before you go to bed, if you wake up in the middle of the night, upon arising before your first meal, etc. At least one quart per day at a minimum. Don't overdo diet sodas and beverages. Anything humans have substituted for the real thing (water) needs to be moderated.

- Bloating can happen in the first few weeks of eating smaller, more frequent meals of real food with real fiber. This is a sign that your digestive system is trying to correct itself and that there is a "traffic jam" in your digestive track. This will go away soon. Just keep eating!

- Dairy products. People often ask at seminars, "what about dairy products?" I recommend eating dairy products, as you can see from the shopping list. If you are lactose intolerant, that is a separate issue. Dairy products are used for different purposes, however, based upon their nutritional profile. For example, I eat non-fat cottage cheese with a little essential oil as one of my "meals". Likewise, I mix non-fat plain yogurt with fresh berries as a "meal". Cheeses I like to use in combination with meals in moderate amounts as a flavor enhancer and the fat helps to satisfy my appetite. I like skim milk, especially with a high fiber breakfast cereal.

- Milk is a healthy food, but high in natural sugars. If you enjoy milk, just pay attention to the protein, fat and carbs and work it into your daily formula. I would consider it a carb food as well as a protein food though due to the sugars, and have it during the early morning/afternoon.

- Protein/fat combinations. In the book, the *"Eskimo Diet"*, the author details how in the meat of most animals in their wild and untamed state is a balance of three parts protein to one part fat. For example, a four-ounce portion of range free buffalo might have about 24 grams of protein and 8 grams of fat. According to the author and a few others I have read, this nutritional make-up can be found in most animals in their natural, undomesticated state. Thus, when we are assembling our own foods, it seems wise to follow this pattern. One of the theories put forth about this naturally occurring protein/fat ratio is that it optimizes the digestion of both nutrients. Optimum digestion is valuable because that improves the utilization of the ingested nutrients by the body. Even if this were not so, it is *still* a good way to keep our fat intake moderate and thought you should know about it. For example, if I were to eat a 4-5 ounce chicken breast (24-27 grams of protein), I would have a slice of cheese with it (8 grams of fat).
- Protein meals before workouts. It is generally recommended that you eat a small protein/fat combination meal 1-2 hours before you workout, unless you workout immediately upon arising. This helps to spare your body from turning to muscle protein for energy as you exercise. Occasionally I will have an orange or something similar before exercising if no suitable protein/fat sources are available, but most of the time I use the Lean Body Latte.
- Carb meals after workouts. After workouts, it is best to have a meal high in carbohydrates to replenish the glycogen stores in your muscles, which were likely tapped into as you worked out. (See Feeding patterns)
- Meal replacement Shakes and bars are o.k. to have on hand for an emergency, but don't overdo them. Real food is *always* best. These products often have numerous ingredients in them, many of which go against the healthier eating grain. Shakes are better than bars though, because they are lower in sugars and fat. These types of products should have at least twenty grams of protein and no more than 10 grams of sugar (under 5 grams is

best). I would not recommend more than one meal replacement bars or shakes per day. The bars especially are tough too digest and can cause bloating and gas, which signals to us that they are not ideal for our bodies. And, do not fall for the whole "net impact" carbs thing. Glycerol is a carbohydrate, no matter how you spell it.

- Throw away or lock up your scale. It is not your friend. Take your focus off of what you weigh and put your focus on your exercise program, and how you feel and look in the mirror. Remember that people who lose weight without building or maintaining muscle simply become smaller, fatter, sicker people (skinny fat people) with less energy and strength and lower metabolisms.

- Put food that may tempt you out of sight. Or better yet, don't buy these types of foods and go out to eat on your junk food night.

- Avoid extremes or exclusiveness. *Almost* all diets and weight loss companies are silly nonsense. Any eating plan that you cannot stay with until they put you six feet under is a waste of time and probably unhealthy.

- Cholesterol. I have never been fully convinced of the whole cholesterol issue as a measure of a person's health, or risk for heart attack. The reasons are that I have watched too many people who obsessively worry about cholesterol, yet at the same time do not exercise, and sometimes even daily drink alcohol, smoke, and for the most part, eat a lot of substandard foods. It just seems pretty harebrained. And, in some cases, I have known fit, strong, active and lean individuals with high cholesterol readings. One has to wonder, which is more dangerous, the cholesterol or the stress of worrying about it. There are, in fact, current studies on whether stress itself actually increases cholesterol. What a vicious cycle that would be! I think cholesterol obviously *should* be paid attention to, but that the real focus should be a lifestyle such as the one you are reading about to reduce the risk of dying prematurely and unnecessarily. In the book, the *Schwarzbein Factor*, Dr. Schwarzbein again does a thorough job of explaining what causes high cholesterol and builds a strong case that it is not caused by eating cholesterol or even high fat foods. Rather, according to her, too much insulin in our systems is what causes high cholesterol.

The causes for this high insulin, according to her, include (but is not limited to) too many refined carbohydrates *in combination* with too little fat. She also wonders why the number of heart attacks has actually been on the increase in this country, even as Americans have reduced their cholesterol intake. Dr. Schwarzbein indicates that the number of deaths from heart attacks has been reduced, but proposes that this is likely due to the improvements in the methods of treating them once they occur. Interestingly, in many of the heart attack deaths, the victim's cholesterol numbers had been within the "safe" zone.

So, concern yourself with cholesterol as you will, but I can't see trying to solve it with yet another pill. People have lived hearty, stalwart, dynamic lives for centuries without all of these pills. Follow this lifestyle, de-stress and live life at its best. Focusing on a number and numbing your body through further medications is not a long-term solution to astonishingly good health. A better solution, before you resort to medications and never having eggs or steak again, is to *thoroughly* follow the lifestyle in this book for one year. At my last checkup, my overall cholesterol was in the outstanding range for a person ten years younger than me, and my HDL's and LDL's were exceptional. This really, really works! And, it can work for you.

- Expect to blow it now and then. The purpose of this lifestyle is not to be neurotic or miserable. No, the purpose is to learn and then live the truth and what works in order to enjoy the benefits of a vibrant healthiness lifestyle. With that in mind, even I sometimes "screw up". Perhaps I will visit somewhere, and they just happen to be serving their world famous lasagna and triple chocolate cheesecake (two of my favorite indulgence foods). Well, because I *LIVE* this lifestyle day in, day out, year after year, and it is an ingrained habit, I can sometimes make an exception to the rules and then get right back on track in an hour or two. If that is not you, then know that for now. But, if you do "blow it", pick yourself right back up and get back in the saddle immediately and move on. It happens. We are, after all, human. When you reach the point where living a fitness lifestyle has become habit for you, then you too can occasionally become a little less disciplined in your eating regimen, and it will not be the end of your healthiness world.

Chapter 19

The People in the

White Coats Are Here!!

"Beware the naked man who offers you his coat."
My Dad

As a kid when one of my friends or I were acting particularly goofy, we would joke that the people in the, "white coats" were going to come and take us away to the funny farm. This image comes to mind sometimes when thinking of what is going on in America with all of the various diet doctors, "nutritionists", and public health officials "weighing in" on how we should eat. If you listen to all of the various arguments put forth, you may find yourself going a little crazy. You have read the formula to successful eating and hope you agree, it is something you can stick with for a lifetime. It will meet all your nutritional requirements, help you to become lean, strong, healthy, and not hurt you in any way.

In listening to nearly all the points of view, it is difficult to agree *completely* with most of them. It seems everyone's "plan" has something of value, but they are also missing the boat in some ways. I would like to take a few moments to personally "weigh in" on some of the more popular diets and nutritional concepts of our time. We will begin by looking at the food guide pyramid, endorsed by countless (but not all) dietitians and our government.

Let me begin by saying, I have the utmost respect for *most* dietitians. While employed at the hospital, I worked with and supervised several dietitians. All of them were professional, followed a fitness lifestyle, and "walked the talk". The same can be said for the many dietitians I have met across the nation, especially those who work in the child nutrition profession in schools across America. It is easy to understand the concern and frustration of dietitians regarding the explosion of various eating plans. These individuals have dedicated their careers to learning and studying the science of nutrition. They must contend with people proclaiming themselves as nutrition experts at every corner, many who propose rather unorthodox methods. Notwithstanding, like all professions, there are good dietitians and some who are not so good. While we may not be able to judge the skill and knowledge of a dietitian, we can with some degree of accuracy judge their ability to get results by talking to and looking at them. I have met several dietitians who are carrying an excessive amount of body fat. It's like a mechanic with a broken down car. Why would someone who can't get his own car working try to tell me how to fix mine?

Some dietitians freely admit that they do absolutely no form of consistent exercise. They state that they just can't find the time, etc, etc. In my opinion, they lack credibility if they are choosing to ignore at least 50% of the healthiness equation. Yet, it is usually these individuals who become most upset when the validity and value of the current food guide pyramid is questioned. Which is where we begin. After we review these diets and nutritional concepts, it will be time to get a little more specific in recommending a daily eating pattern *for the majority* of people in this nation.

The Food Guide Pyramid

(The earth is flat, no one will ever run a three minute mile, and yours is not to question why)

Over the past few decades, the phrase "think out of the box" has become increasingly common. Most of us would agree that this concept has been useful and is needed in order to get the best results. Conversely, insanity has been defined as continuing to do the same thing and hoping to get different results. Let's keep those concepts in mind as we proceed. My experience has been that questioning the foundational principles of the Food Guide Pyramid can quickly make you unpopular. About a year ago, I was working as part of a task force on childhood obesity. There were about 18 people on the task force, from various sectors of society who are involved in influencing the education and lives of children.

When the subject of nutrition education came up, I questioned whether or not we were going to continue teaching the food guide pyramid as it doesn't seem to be effective in helping people become lean and fit. The reaction I received verged on venomous. People who previously were kind and smiling soon began to glare and fume. How dare suggest that this pillar of academia, constructed by the countries finest researchers and scientists could be flawed? No, I was quickly told, the problem is not in the pyramid itself, but rather in people's interpretation of it. Oh, really?

Doesn't anyone else wonder why we have seen a marked increase in obesity since the inception of the food guide pyramid concept in the mid 1980's? Just this week, the Center of Disease control released a study on obesity in America. This is what they found: over the last thirty years, the caloric intake of all Americans has increased, including men and women, but more significantly with women. They also stated that calorie intake was found to have come primarily from . . . carbohydrates. No, I am not suggesting that everyone run over to Atkins. The suggestion is however, that the Food Guide pyramid is flawed. Atkins and the others will be perused momentarily, but to deny the positive results that those types of plans have provided seems like sticking ones head in the sand. It seems wise to examine the possibility of combining the best of Atkins (and similar lower carb concepts) with the best of the Food Guide Pyramid. Perhaps there is something to be learned from both. I don't agree with everything about the Atkins plan, but must give it some credit for showing that Americans eat way too many carbohydrates, especially refined, processed, sweetened, and "fake" ones.

The food guide pyramid, on the other hand, places *WAY* too much emphasis on breads and grains, not enough on fresh vegetables, fresh whole fruits, lean proteins, and adequate amounts of *natural* fats. Even the categories themselves are questionable. The categories on dairy products, fruits and vegetables are reasonable. However, there should be more emphasis on vegetables over fruits because most people seem to do o.k. eating fruit, but struggle when it comes to vegetables. Vegetables are of incredible value in regards to nutrients and fiber. Bottled and canned juices should not qualify as a fruit because most of the commercial juices are extremely high in simple sugars. Remember; eat real foods as close as possible to their natural state! I know that I am not making a whole lot of friends by saying some of these things, but if we are trying to become lean, fat-incinerating, anti-aging, wellness machines, we have to tighten things up a bit.

Breads and cereals should be replaced with a category called, "natural complex carbohydrates". This would include whole grain brown rice, peas, corn, beans, baked and boiled potatoes, and on occasion (once per day is sufficient, twice per day maximum) 100% whole grain, naturally high fiber, unsweetened bread products such as a sandwich bread or cereal. Yes, I know that many people would turn up their noses at some of these suggestions, but it would be difficult to argue that these foods are not among the best choices for complex carbohydrates. And the best should be our goal. The current recommended 6-11 servings of bread/grains per day is extreme and a sure contributor to fatness. Trying to change that specific recommendation is no easy task, as it helps to fatten the pockets of the major cereal makers (you know who they are) and powerful lobby groups such as wheat growing associations.

This raises an issue that many of us may not be aware of. There is serious money surrounding the food guide pyramid and how it is constructed. To change it would require changing what is taught in the universities, colleges, and schools across America. That would mean changing books, promotional materials, etc. But the real issue is the various special interest groups who stand to either benefit or be harmed by what the federal government and health authorities recommend. Just ask the egg and beef industries. They have taken a serious hit over the last two decades, due perhaps to knee jerk reactions regarding the potential harms from their products.

There are dietitians who agree with many of these issues; yet not many speaking up publicly. Recently however, I read an editorial response from a registered dietitian in *Fitness Management* magazine. Interestingly, the dietitian is also a certified health and fitness instructor with the American College of Sports Medicine. He states that, "For many years dietitians have embraced the food pyramid. While it is true that they have promoted fruits and vegetables, they have also pushed the consumption of pasta, cereals, bagels and breads. The average American has consumed excessive quantities of these refined sugars for many years already. How long have we been told to increase intake of fruits and vegetables to at least five daily? Research consistently demonstrates that these are the two healthiest food groups. So why don't they make up the base of the pyramid?" He goes on to say, "the U.S. Department of Agriculture was the managing organization for the development of the pyramid. Is it possible that this group had any influence in placing its interests in the base of the pyramid? The answer will be a definitive yes if any carbohydrates are recommended in the same quantities as fruits and vegetables in the forthcoming pyramid. Is it impossible to assemble a group of scientific, unbiased, non-industry-associated individuals to construct the next pyramid? Maybe consumers would finally benefit more than food manufacturers who don't care at all about public health". I concur with most of this dietitian's opinion and assertive words.

Still, I am a capitalist and understand the need to make a living. Farmers and the agricultural industry are a foundation of this country. But it does seem askew that a few powerful groups can influence what is considered good for us to fuel our bodies with. By the way, the Fit Food Eating Formula greatly supports the agricultural and farming industries on the whole. Eating a variety of real, "natural state" foods that you can either pick, pull from the ground, milk or catch benefits America's farms.

Schools are under the microscope for being a contributor to the growing obesity of America's youth. To be sure, the schools could do a better job. To their credit, many of the schools *are* improving their menus and offerings. Despite the flaws of the current guidelines, many school food service programs are improving students nutritional health *within the current guidelines* by providing the **best** choices from each of the food groups defined by the pyramid. By offering the opportunity to have fresh vegetables and fruits, along with an array of other healthy, tasteful and attractive foods, we are making a positive inroad.

Poor health, fitness and obesity are an individual responsibility and a societal issue. It really needs to start with each one of us as adults and parents, and then taught to the youth at the same time. Remember, couch potatoes have simply bred, "Tator tots" in most cases. I find it interesting that so many (not all) of the critics of school foods are often people who are unfit themselves, do not exercise, eat a substandard diet, and even smoke. These behavioral issues do not make them "bad" people, of course. It just calls into question whether or not they are qualified to speak on issues of healthiness. If they, as intelligent, experienced and educated adults have not been able to discipline themselves or figure out how to become lean and fit, how can they expect others or younger people to do so?

As stated, the tide at schools *is* beginning to turn more in the direction of what I and others familiar with fitness and fit foods recommend. Less refined, human made foods, more vegetables, fruits, lean proteins and natural fats are available. In the Dover school system (New Hampshire) for example, the nutrition department is now serving "bun less" burgers, hot dogs and chicken patties. According to administrator Mark Covell, "they are cutting out the roll and just giving them the protein". Now, if they can teach the students about body composition and the value of muscle, we are really making progress!

Let's get back to the current food guide pyramid. The current food guide pyramid was probably designed with good intentions. And yes, a rare few who follow it closely and do 30-45 minutes of aerobic exercise every day are able to stay "thin" and appear fit. But this does not hold true for the majority of people. It is time for a change. Even the Harvard University School of Public Health and others are proposing changes. Unfortunately, what I have seen so far does not look too impressive. One of the proposed new pyramids from Harvard looks like a vegetarian wrote it. Vegetarianism is a whole other subject. It may not be a bad idea to actually build a guide just for vegetarians that insures they are getting all the nutrients they require, especially complete proteins.

If the Pyramid does not change to something more middle of the road, though, people will continue to look for better answers. Which brings us to the seemingly now everywhere and widely worshipped Atkins diet.

Atkins Diet

The Atkins diet has been around for several decades now. It was developed and promoted by the now deceased Dr. Robert Atkins. These days, it is at perhaps its highest point of popularity ever. It is seen daily on the Internet, television commercials and more and more restaurants across the country. Dr. Atkins, as mentioned, should be credited with showing America that they eat too many refined carbohydrates. To their credit, the Atkins Company has now come up with the, "New Atkins" diet, which includes more vegetables with meals. Still, Atkins has gone way too far in regards to fat consumption. The idea that we eat too many refined carbs and have reduced fat consumption too low is sound reasoning. But to go so far in the other direction makes little good sense. My formula keeps fat at about 27% of calories consumed, which is enough to receive the benefits of fat, while reducing potential dangers of too much.

Because I consider myself to be a research scientist, I usually don't just join a bandwagon of critics without some legitimate experimentation. Usually I simply use myself as the test subject! So, I tried Atkins for a period of about two months. As a result, I did lose weight. In fact, quite a bit. Unfortunately, I also lost energy and a significant portion of muscle even thought I was strength training. Perhaps the most noted drawback though, were the changes I noticed in my digestive processes. I will spare you the details here, but it was obvious too me that things were not working in a comfortable and regular fashion in my stomach and intestines. Maybe now that Atkins is stressing more vegetables, digestion could be enhanced for some.

But the REAL problem with Atkins is this. It is a *DIET.* Or should I say, a diet only! Almost everyone you meet who is on Atkins is not exercising at the same time. They are simply people who are too lazy to actually embrace a fitness lifestyle. They are looking for the fast and easy way to drop weight. Atkins makes virtually no effort to stress the need for exercise, and when it is mentioned, it is extremely vague. And this was a doctor?? Why is this? Because mentioning exercise or getting specific about it would scare off those who only want to be passive and diet. Thus, as we discussed, those who follow Atkins, lose a significant amount of muscle and become *smaller fatter people*. Nearly everyone I meet who has lost noticeable weight on Atkins, without a concern for muscle, end up looking like a sickly, weak, unfit bag of bones. They do not look fit, lean, strong and healthy. Now, there are always exceptions, but this is the rule, rather than the exception.

It is interesting that Dr. Atkins was always seen in a white coat. In fact, most of the rashes of diet doctors trying to cash in on the obesity plague are usually seen in white coats. Are they perhaps, the people in the white coats mentioned at the beginning of this chapter? What are they trying to cover up? If their methods are so great in helping us to become lean and fit, why don't they show us what they look like in a t-shirt at least? No, I don't think they need to pose in a pair of Calvin Klein's, but it would be more convincing to see that they are actually lean. There are a couple of these diet doctors, who to their credit are emphasizing specific types of exercise in their programs. These include the authors of *The Schwarzbein Principle* and the authors of *Protein Power*. I will review their programs momentarily. Unfortunately for them, it seems that by mentioning exercise in their programs they are hurting their popularity and profitability. Perhaps that is o.k. with them. Maybe their motive is not simply to become rich and famous, but rather to offer people a plan that will positively impact their health.

South Beach Diet

The latest player in the diet doctor field is the south beach diet. To his credit, the author of this book, Dr. Arthur Agatston is one smart "diet cookie." It seems that he was able to see the benefits of Atkins concept, but realized it was too extreme to receive much positive press. Thus, he wisely modified it, gave it a sexy name and put an aqua blue cover on the book to help us feel like we were actually at the ocean. The marketing is brilliant, without a doubt. And, in truth, his eating plans sound more reasonable than Atkins. So far, I haven't seen a whole lot wrong with it in regards to its long-term recommendations, with one rather large exception. The good Doctor clearly states in his marketing, **NO EXERCISE REQUIRED**. This is a joke. He calls himself a cardiologist, and then says no exercise required. Earlier I said he was wise. Well, this aspect of his plan is not wise, but crafty. Of course, he assures, "no exercise required", otherwise his chances of becoming rich and famous from the diet-only crowd will be "slim to none"!

By the way, does being a cardiologist make one a health and fitness expert? To me, using your cardiologist status as credentials to being an expert on leanness, fitness and health is like a mechanic who claims to know how to win the Indy 500, yet has never personally raced or actually helped anyone else win the race. Just because one knows how to fix a broken car does not mean one knows how to operate it at its highest performing level. I have heard that cardiologists suffer a greater percentage of heart attacks than the rest of the population, so they may not be the best source of fitness advice. In fact, the most prominent cardiologist in my hometown was known to smoke up to three packs of cigarettes per day. If your cardiologist is lean, fit, strong and healthy, then they can probably give some good instruction as they are living out the lifestyle themselves. But if they themselves are not the model of stellar leanness and healthiness, you might seek out a better mechanic!

But, no doubt, Dr, Argen has been able to parlay his cardiologist background into financial success with his south beach diet. And why not, as the south beach diet states you will lose 8-10 pounds off your belly in the first 2 weeks. Well of course you will! If you cut out all carbs which reduces calories (ala Atkins) for a period of time, especially when you have been eating way too many refined carbs and related junk, you will quickly drop a lot of water weight, some fat and muscle to boot. Atkins does the same thing. I know some people are having success with the ocean blue book, or whatever it's called. I am just appalled that this guy calls himself a cardiologist without feeling any guilt about excluding exercise. Take off your white jacket, good doctor, and shows us the leanness.

The Schwarzbein Principle

On a more positive note, this is a book I think everyone should read. The author, a doctor whose training was in endocrinology and metabolism, does a good job of explaining why high-carb, low fat eating regimens do not work. She also reviews cholesterol, pointing out that its relationship to heart attacks is largely misunderstood. As stated previously, many people with good cholesterol numbers suffer and die from heart attacks while many with supposedly bad, high cholesterol numbers do not. In addition, she explains why eating foods high in cholesterol is not how cholesterol numbers become elevated, rather excess carbohydrates are the cause.

The author is in favor of eating real, natural, unprocessed foods, lowering overall carbohydrate intake, eliminating all stimulants, and makes a point of emphasizing an exercise lifestyle. From what I could see, she is rather vague on her exercise recommendations, which is a drawback of this book. Dr. Schwarzbein is also an advocate for hormone replacement therapy. I am of course, less qualified than she on this matter. Still, I have read of experiments where hormone replacement therapy can be avoided through an effective exercise and lifestyle program that includes strength training.

Protein Power

The authors of protein power have advocated a higher protein, low carbohydrate regimen for many years now. Their program seems to be better balanced than Atkins, with less fat and more vegetables. Personally, I think it is still too low in carbohydrates. What I like about these authors, though, is that they are not strictly, "Diet Doctors". Perhaps because of their exercise inclusion, they have not experienced the same success as the strictly cash motivated competition. They, like me, advocate strength training as the best form of exercise for getting the best results. They, however, promote a "super slow" method of strength training, which has been proven highly effective. I have referenced their book in the appendix, if you are interested in learning more of this method. While this "super slow" is effective, most people have difficulty staying with it. It requires very intense effort, which can be difficult to sustain over a long period of time.

Weight Watchers

Weight watchers was discussed at length in an earlier chapter. Some people seem to like weight watchers, and if it works for you, great. What I think they could do better is to emphasize effective exercise and drop their reliance on over processed, additive filled packaged meals. Their point counting system is their trademark, so it is doubtful they would ever drop that method. Still, it makes better sense (to me at least) to teach people the nutritional basics of food in order to give them greater independence. If you choose to follow weight watchers, you should most definitely strength train properly and consistently, and you will have much better odds of getting real, healthy, and permanent improvements.

Suzanne Somers

Suzanne Somers has written many books on her diet approach. First off, I have to say that I have difficulty trusting anyone who could sell and make millions on something like the, "Thigh Master". The thigh master qualifies as fitness "magic dust". Suzanne is currently busy promoting another piece of plastic fitness equipment on infomercials that also can join the parade of promise makers and breakers when it comes to a lean, fit body.

Her eating plans are a combination of low-carb and food separation. Some critic's question whether she actually originated these concepts, or simply borrowed them from others and then meshed them into her own words. I have reviewed her plans and see nothing too out of kilter in them in regards to eating. Many people, myself included, have utilized others ideas as well as their own in coming up with an effective eating plan. I do not fault her for that. In addition, I have even met a few people who lost some excess body fat following her plans. But here's the kicker. Those who did lose fat and were able to do so in a permanent fashion, followed an exercise program similar to the one I teach. They did weight lifting coupled with endurance and aerobic exercise. They did not use thigh masters or any of Suzanne's other plastic "pipe dream" machines. If Suzanne would include effective exercise plans in her diet books, she could help a lot more people.

Body for Life

Bill Phillips, the author of Body for Life, has helped thousands become lean and fit. He deserves credit for bringing the benefits of weight lifting/ bodybuilding to the general public. In truth, I am a little envious that I did not think of his approach myself. He has become hugely successful through his book, magazines and supplement company. His program works. If you are at all unfit, over fat, weak etc, and you follow his programs, you will have a high degree of success. His workout regimen is similar to that used by bodybuilders for decades. A combination of strength training, higher intensity aerobic exercise and smaller, more frequent meals made up of higher proteins, moderate healthy carbs and low fat. Again, it will work for you. And no, you won't end up looking like a pro bodybuilder.

Notwithstanding, I feel his workouts take too long. You can accomplish the same results in about two-thirds to half the time with more effective workouts. Also, he unashamedly promotes his protein meal replacement throughout all his books. His products are good quality, and can be effective, but at the same time are expensive. They are also unnecessary. By following what I recommend, you can get the same (or better) health and fitness results eating real, less expensive foods. He states that his meal replacements aren't needed for success. Yet he continues to use direct and subliminal suggestion throughout all of his materials to hint at the success you might miss without his meals in a packet. Every sample day meal pattern he shows includes *three* of his meal replacements. If you want to spend the rest of your life spending hundreds each month on meal replacement shakes, and an extra hour or more each week exercising, then his plan may be for you.

Diets, Diets, Diets, etc

No doubt, they're are many I have missed, and many more to come. You are, by now, hopefully better armed to evaluate any nutritional program that comes along. Just keep the following in mind. If a plan does not emphasize exercise, and especially exercise that builds or maintains muscle, it automatically disqualifies itself. Still, if a nutritional plan is sound in its foundation, you can simply combine it with either my exercise program, or one similar, and have good success.

I may be repeating myself, but some things can't be overemphasized. *Do not diet without exercising.* Eat adequate amounts of lean proteins. Include some high calcium foods each day. Eat lots of high fiber green vegetables and fresh fruits, especially unsweetened berries. Eat at least 50-100 grams of carbs each day. Get them from natural sources. The less human altered the better. To stay lean, eat your carbs before 5:00 pm. Eat adequate natural fats, about one ounce per meal with about 4 of your daily meals. Eat 5-8 smaller, equally sized meals per day. Reduce stimulants and artificial beverages as much as possible. Drink more water.

Yes, that is rather general info, but if any plan you are considering does not include the above, I would proceed with caution.

Food Guide Pyramid versus the Fit-Food Formula Fortress

In order to show that what I recommend is not TOO far off from the USDA Food Guide Pyramid, it seemed wise to quickly review what the pyramid recommends. After that, I will introduce, in a somewhat similar format, the, "Fit-Food Formula Fortress." This is my version of how most of us should feed and fortify our bodies and our health. First, we will review the current pyramid.

The Food Guide Pyramid says to daily have:

- **Fats, oils and sweets sparingly.** The problem here is that (1) *very low fat* diets don't work (2) sparingly is way too wide of a guideline.
- **Milk, Yogurt, cheeses.** (2-3 servings per day). My concept is similar, in that I too recommend 2-3 servings of dairy per day, but primarily in lean form as the main segment of a meal. For example, non-fat or low fat cottage cheese with essential fatty acid oil or non-fat yogurt with fresh whole fruits. Cheeses are recommended in smaller amounts (one/ one and a half ounces, 7-15 grams fat) as meal enhancers such as in omelets, with a salad, etc.
- **Meat, poultry, beans, nuts.** (4-6 servings per day). Again, my concept is similar, in that I recommend 4-6 servings of lean protein per day. Beans, however, are more of a carbohydrate, and thus are moved to the complex carb category. Nuts and seeds have been given their own category, as they are nutritious, yet high in fats with a moderate amount of protein and carbs.
- **Fruit.** (2-4 servings per day). I recommend the same, but specifically recommend more of the higher fiber berries.
- **Vegetables.** (3-5 servings per day). I recommend the same, with the exception of the more complex carb vegetables such as corn and peas, and move them instead into the complex carb category.
- **Bread, cereal, rice, bagels.** (6-11 servings daily). This is where we primarily differ. The category I have replaced it with is "complex carbs". I recommend only 1-3 servings per day. Primarily from un-mechanized, non-enhanced, or processed sources. This is enough to satisfy all nutritional needs and energy levels for nearly every person in this country. If a person, such as a competitive athlete, etc were still hungry after eating what I recommend, they could have an additional serving or two of complex carbs, but I still feel they would be better off eating *natural* corn, beans or baked skin-on potatoes rather than human made cereal and bread products.

In totality, the Food Guide Pyramid recommends between 14-29 servings per day. It is based on a 2000 calorie per day intake. I have devised my own "guide". It is, in my opinion, what we should be recommending for the majority of Americans. As I write this, it is April 2004. It will be interesting to see how the "new" Food Guide Pyramid compares to what I recommend. My "Fortress" below suggests between 18-24 servings/portions per day, and recommended calories are based on a sliding scale of a person's ideal lean bodyweight and active muscle building activities.

By the way, a fortress is something you could actually live in and with, whereas a pyramid would be a difficult place to take up residence. If everyone in America ate according to this formula, we would see dramatic improvements in health and fitness and *inconceivable* reductions in health care costs.

The Fit-Food Formula Fortress . . .
Making mansions of mighty good health!

Exercise. This is the foundation of the formula, and without it you are building your health future on quicksand. In order for the rest of the formula to function properly, you must fulfill this step. Otherwise, there is no sense in progressing. Include at least two-three days of strength training exercise each week, and add endurance/bodyweight exercises and aerobic exercise on non-strength training days.

Complex Clean (unrefined) Carbohydrates—(2-3 portions daily.) Portions would be 2-4 ounces or a handful. This includes all beans, long grain brown rice, corn, peas, baked or boiled potatoes, 100% whole *no added sugar* grain breads/cereals.

Fruits. (2-4 portions) Fresh whole fruits. Especially focus on blueberries, strawberries and blackberries, etc. They are high in fiber. Also include plenty of citrus fruits such as oranges and kiwi.

Fats. (Approximately four 1 to 1.5 ounce portions per day). Use natural sources, both unsaturated and some saturated. I usually try to get 2/3 of my fat calories from unsaturated, and 1/3 from saturated. Include oils, cheeses, avocados, real mayonnaise, etc.

Lean Proteins. (4-6 portions daily, 2-6 ounces each). Try to include 2-3 from low /no-fat calcium sources such as low fat cottage cheese, whey protein or non-fat plain yogurt.

Vegetables. (4-6 portions daily, approximately ½ cup or a small handful. For you veggie haters, a little is better than nothing!) Try to include some veggies with at least 4 of your meals. I try to always have a little fresh spinach, bell peppers, or broccoli florets handy.

Nuts, Nut Butters, or Seeds. (1 portion daily). A portion will be about ¼-1/3 cup or one to three slightly rounded tablespoons. Again, use as natural as possible of sources, no oils added, etc. It is suggested that nuts, nut butters or seeds are eaten alone as one of your meals.

Junk Food Night (JFN)—eat or drink anything and as much as you want, designated day each week, 1-4 hour period depending upon your current condition. My JFN is almost always Friday evening, from about 5:00 pm—9:00 p.m. We do *suggest* that you use *some* discipline and not binge, but rather slowly *enjoy* & savor the foods you like to occasionally indulge in and satisfy those cravings.

This "fortress" is offered as an alternative to the USDA Food Guide Pyramid. The USDA is currently considering updating the pyramid, but until then I wanted to offer the best formula I know of. I believe it addresses the inadequacies of the pyramid, Atkins, and other "diets". But in order to achieve *maximum* results, I suggest *progressively implementing* all of the, "21 Principles of Becoming a Lean, Fat-Incinerating, Anti-Aging Machine" found on pages 212-214.

Lean Body Latte'
"A muscle making 'miracle mix' of morning magnificence!"

This can be your breakfast! Do not turn your nose up without trying this. Many initial scoffers have become die-hard addicts to this rich, creamy, delicious and nutritious concoction. For the best results, drink immediately upon waking up. This is also good to have 1 hour to 30 minutes before your workout.

1) Make a cup of Coffee. Regular or Decaf.

2) In a large mug, place one or two scoops of "instantized" (mixes easily) whey protein powder. Most whey proteins come with a scoop. The brand I use has 23 grams of protein per scoop. Most women will want to use one scoop (23 grams) and most men; two scoops (46 grams). Most whey proteins are flavored, such as chocolate, vanilla, etc. My personal favorite flavor for mixing with coffee is cocoa-mochaccino from Champion Nutrition. Use a fork to stir the whey in. Stir for a minute or two and mash any extra against the side of the mug to break up any that has not dissolved and make it smooth and creamy.

3) Next you will add Heavy Whipping Cream. (You may leave the cream out, and the taste and nutrient content will still be excellent. I suggest at least *trying* the cream though) Use only *real* heavy whipping cream, plain and simple, no anything added. The amount of cream you use will depends upon how much whey protein you use. The idea is to have a 3 to 1 ratio of protein to fat. For example, if you use one scoop of whey (23 gms), you would use 1/3 as many fat grams or about 7.66 grams of fat, which is approximately 1.5 tablespoons of cream. Check to see how much fat, if any, the whey protein has before you add the cream. This drink will satisfy your hunger, and provides essential protein and fat.

4) I also add one tablespoon of Benefiber. This is a fiber supplement that is tasteless and undetectable. I would suggest you do the same, although that of course, is optional.

You can buy whey at any health food store, and I believe Costco is now carrying it. I do offer whey protein on my web site at *www.fitfooddude.com*. Enjoy your healthy new breakfast alternative. For more information on whey protein and its benefits, visit *www.wheyoflife.org*.

In order to improve your chances of success, it is important to keep track of your food intake, especially for the first four weeks. I have been keeping track of food intake for decades now, and intend to do so for the rest of my life. This only takes me a few moments a day. I simply jot down at the top of my daily planner when and what I had for my first feeding, second feeding, etc. This is a habit I recommend you form, as it will help you to form better health and thus a brighter future. If you would like to see a sample of the kind of chart I use, go to my website www.fitfooddude.com. You are welcome to download and print my Daily Nutrition Log for your personal use.

Section VII

**Get You're Head Together . . . .
Because You Can't Get Very
Far With Out It!**

Chapter 20

The Delivering Dozen . . .

The United Nations of Healthiness

*"The good Lord gave you a body that can stand most
anything. It's your mind you have to convince"*

Vince Lombardi

One of the most common instructions from coaches in the world
of sports is that "the body will go where the head takes it." In the
realm of lifestyle change, and especially with exercise, your success
in making a permanent improvement will start and end in the
mind. Even with all of the best information and resources on the
planet, none of us will be able to accomplish anything significant
or long term unless our mind tells our body to do something, and
then to keep doing it over and over. It may be then, that flexing
the muscle between your ears is going to be your greatest challenge.
We will have to learn to pump up our motivation, enthusiasm and
confidence in order to pulverize procrastination, self-doubt, and
fears.

Many of us need to get better at managing our minds and thoughts. Of course, this is much easier said than done. Throughout history, the complexities of the mind, emotions, and will have been one of the dominating themes of study and debate. Theologians, philosophers, and psychologists have pondered and continue to ponder what makes us tick, and why we behave as we do.

Borrowing from what others have taught in the past in combination with my own insights gleaned from training others, some noteworthy tools and thoughts will be shared on how you can "start and stay the healthiness course". These 'tools" have been set up into a structure similar to the obstacles that opened the book. You may recall that the book began with a description of the "Deceptive Dozen". It is time now to move towards a more optimistic and encouraging approach: hence I would like to introduce the "Delivering Dozen". These are twelve qualities of character hopefully taught to us throughout our lifetime. They are a *stronger* force than the deceptive dozen, and when called upon consistently, can overcome the deceptive dozen. They are not new, but unfortunately in these days where "comfort is king" and the quest is for easy living, they are not all that common. They can, however, be supremely powerful forces.

The "Delivering Dozen" will also be referred to as my "nations". Yes, my nations. Hillary had her village; I have my "nations". I have discovered that it takes *nations* to raise a life of healthiness. Thus, I have formed a fitness coalition of "united nations ". This is a force of stalwart mental focus friends to help us counter the assault on our healthiness. These nations are brave, loyal, and always there for you when you need them. I trust you will find them to be of great value as you fight the good fight for your fitness future. Always keep in mind that the *real* struggle begins and ends in our mind, with our thoughts, ideas, and attitudes. It is time for more of us to embrace these qualities and principles, not only for enhancing our health and fitness, but also for buttressing our individual futures in general, and the futures of those who will follow us. These qualities, characteristics, or whatever one would choose to call them, are the "recipe" for success no matter the field of endeavor.

A few years ago, I did a seminar in my hometown. Several community members, friends, and co-workers eagerly attended. Perhaps some merely came to offer me support and encouragement, but several were hoping that this was going to be the big "AHA" for them. They hoped that I would provide them with the "secrets" and motivation they needed to initiate a health and fitness revolution in their lives. A few of them expressed such hopes to me before the event. After the seminar, these same folks said that the information was terrific and delivered in a way to get them excited about moving in the right direction. Yet, a follow-up done after six months revealed that only a *very* small percentage of those in attendance had done anything with the life transforming tools they were given. I have seen this happen time and again, all around the country. Yes, it is true that my skill and effectiveness in presenting could be a factor. But after several years of presenting, though I can always improve, I am certain that the method and content are not the primary problem. The people in the audiences are not the problem either. The audiences I speak to are made up of smart, hard working, well-intentioned individuals. The problem is that intelligence and good intentions aren't enough.

How can we win this fight that sometimes goes on between our ears? You know, the little voices that tell us things like, "you deserve to sleep in . . . I'm too old for this . . . this will never work, etc., etc.". Scripture tells us "we are transformed (changed) by the *renewing* of our minds". Zig Ziglar, the famous motivational speaker says, that, "we are what we are, we are where we are, because of what has *gone into* our minds, we change what we are, we change where we are, by changing what *goes into* our minds. You may have heard that the mind is like a computer. If you put bad information into a computer, bad information comes out. The term used to describe this reality is, "Garbage in, garbage out". Let's agree now to take out the garbage that may have stunk up our past fitness pursuits. Instead, we will begin sweeping our minds clean in order to make room for the Delivering Dozen, the united nations of our new and improved health and fitness lifestyle.

The nations below will have some unavoidable crossover or similarities in their content. Still, I have tried to put them in the order in which I find they naturally fall. Follow them like all else in this book. That is, progressively, consistently and diligently. Read this section several times, to see which n-ations could help your mindset the most. Find a way to put some of the concepts below into your memory bank a little each day. Even five minutes of reading in this area each day can add up over time. The clock is ticking. It is time to start **immediately**, and progress brick by brick, little by little, each and every day. Because the fight that goes on between our ears can be relentless, it will likely require a relentless approach on our parts to reach the shore of triumphant healthiness.

The Delivering Dozen: a coalition of twelve nations.

I. Initi-ation.

> *"Those who initiate change will have a better opportunity to manage the change that is inevitable."*
> William Pollard

> *"Vision without action is hallucination."*
> Don Clifton

> *"Life is too short, and the time we waste in yawning can never be regained."*
> Stendahl

"Focus on changing behavior before attitude. We don't think ourselves into a new way of acting, we act our way into new ways of thinking". After some reflecting, I've come to believe that this statement is only *half* true. Instead, attitude needs to be addressed *at the same time* as the actions. Whatever you do though, don't wait until you *feel* like it to get started. That is the sure sign of future failure. Countless people have contacted me to tell me how much they learned from and enjoyed my presentation/seminar. Then, I will run into them a year later, and often they *still* have not taken any action on what they learned. In the conversations that follow, they invariably express their intention to get started . . ."as soon as . . . when . . . if only". While it seems these folks are sincere, their thinking runs counter to nearly every principle of success. As discussed in chapter one of this book, the book, *Think and Grow Rich*, by Napoleon Hill, offers twelve principles of success. The principle I remember most is that successful people make big decisions quickly, and then change them slowly. Those who live lives of continual failure (inability to reach goals) make big decisions slowly, and then change them quickly and often. There are only a few decisions in your lifetime bigger than the one to take better care of yourself. You have a literal *goldmine* of health, fitness and wellness information in your hands with this book. Start using it today and your mental attitude will toughen as your body strengthens.

II. Destin-ation.

> *"Vision is the art of seeing things invisible"*
> Jonathan Swift

> *"Have a vision. Be demanding."*
> Colin Powell

> *"We are limited, not by our abilities, but by our vision."*
> Anonymous

Where do you want to end up? How do you want to end up? There are many things out of our control. Conversely, there are many things over which we have a degree of control or ability to influence. Thinking about our ultimate destination is something that we can take part in. Proverbs says, "Without a vision, the people perish". That is, if a person has no destination in mind, then any kind of living will do. Look around you. Do you see any people "perishing" due to lack of health and fitness? When I talk about perishing, I am not saying these folks go, "poof" and vanish into thin air. Rather they slowly progress downward until they are living a life that does not become all that it could have been. And this is exactly what is happening to the health and fitness of the majority of Americans. A business associate told me that he recently returned from a trip to Europe and Asia and that he found it almost embarrassing when he returned to the states. As he made his way through the airport, he couldn't help but notice the difference in the level of fitness from the countries he had just left. Many of these countries have far less than we do materially, yet the people are in better shape physically. In his words, the difference was shocking. Perhaps our lives have become too easy.

What do you envision for your life? Do you have any highly motivating dreams? What do you want to pass on to your kids and grandkids? You and I have far more influence than we realize, for good or for bad. If you have a concrete, value filled, powerful vision or dream you are going to want to be in stellar shape and condition, because you have a destiny to fulfill, a destination to reach. There is no room for whining, wimpy soft excuses (well, maybe once in a while, just don't make it a habit). No lying in bed feeling sorry for our selves or cutting ourselves slack *day after day after day after day*. Figure out what you want for your destination or destiny. Remember you are influencing not just your life, but also those around you and for generations to come. Resolve to reach your destination. Get a little fire in your eyes and hunger in your belly. We can rest when we are dead. We are going to be dead much longer than we will be alive. Life is for the living.

If you don't have a destination in mind, you should seriously think about it. A study was done several years ago with regard to dreams. In the study, participants were allowed to fall asleep, but as soon as they entered the "dream state", they were awakened. This went on for several days, and as it did the participants first became lethargic, then depressed, then very irritable and were on the verge of becoming violent when the experiment was stopped. One of the conclusions drawn from the experiment was that without a dream or vision (a worthy *destination* in mind), a person is on the slow road to insanity. I am convinced that there is a clear connection between having a destiny in mind and taking care of our selves in order to reach the goal. We have always been told that, "failing to plan is planning to fail". Recently I heard it said that, "planning to fail ahead, is planning to fail in the future". You and I want brighter, fitter futures. Get a clear, specific and well-defined vision of that destination today.

III. Inspir-ation.

> *"Method is much, technique is much, but inspiration is even more."*
>
> > Benjamin Cardoza

> *"You can't wait for inspiration. You have to go after it with a club."*
>
> > Jack London

> *"No one was ever great without some portion of divine inspiration."*
>
> > Marcus Tullius Cicero

What inspires you? What are you passionate about? This issue is close to the dream issue just mentioned but it's not exactly the same. Inspiration plays a key role in our ability to become and stay self-disciplined. A factor that separates the haves from the have-not's, the winners from the losers in the pursuit of healthiness, is self-discipline. And self-discipline is usually born of a strong inspiration that moves you, *even* when you don't feel like moving. For millions of people, their inspiration is primarily appearance focused. That is, they simply want to look good. People are reconstructing their appearance in many creative and expensive ways these days. One of the problems with this is that their health does not always benefit from these "makeovers". Thus, if you are going to be successful over the long haul, in good times and bad, a deeper inspiration than merely improving our outward looks is something we need to discover and cling to.

As many of us mature, we begin to become less concerned with the focus on appearance, and seek to be fully alive and thrive, while loving others and making a positive difference in the world. With that in mind, we would be wise to identify what *inspires* rather than tires us in our pursuit of healthiness. If we don't, our efforts may expire when we encounter the inevitable bumps in the road. For example, many people are able to get started on a new and improved healthiness path and begin making progress. As long as life is running smoothly they continue. The struggle begins when life is not smooth for whatever reason. Perhaps they did not sleep well, they're feeling a little under the weather, they've been up all night with a child or they've had a stressful day at work. When life gets tough, following through on efforts that call for self-discipline becomes a real challenge.

A comment often heard is "I wish I had more self-discipline". Many of those who make this statement then go on to express how much they admire others with self-discipline. They make these statements as if it were something unattainable for them. This of course is untrue, as it is simply a mindset, anyone can choose to adopt. In my case, self-discipline has developed out of a strong desire to live a successful life, coupled with days, months and years of choosing to pursue a healthy lifestyle. This choice has helped to create a relentless determination to squeeze more out of this grand opportunity to live. I imagine others who have the discipline habit have similar goals. To live a life of less than what is within our reach has never made sense, and the older I get, the less sense it makes.

One of the reasons that I focused on self-discipline is that the successful people I have studied and known possess this quality. They do not concern themselves with what everyone else is doing or not doing. Rather, they find out what works for them, and what does not. Then, they do more of what does work, and less of what does not, and focus on the former until it becomes a habit in their lives. We can do the same with healthiness.

For example, even when I go on vacation I like to wake up earlier than everyone else and work out. The work out I do when traveling is usually just bodyweight calisthenics, 15 minutes in length, and perhaps not as intense as normal. But, it is enough to keep me in the habit of training, stimulates my muscles and heart, and creates the endorphin effect. As a result, I feel really good and approach my day with more optimism and energy. I have found that if I sleep in and don't work out, I tend to feel a bit sluggish and less enthusiastic.

Oftentimes I think to myself, "You know, you *are* on vacation. Maybe you should just relax and enjoy yourself. Most people don't work out on their vacation". Through trial and error, though, I have learned that getting my butt out of bed and exercising works much better for me, and probably you as well. It is definitely a better choice for my life, even though there ARE days when I FEEL like sleeping in a little. In 99 out of 100 cases though, if I get up and get moving I am quite happy that I did within moments.

Similar challenges and temptations to break from self-discipline will hit you at inopportune moments. The company picnic or the family BBQ is usually one of those times. You will have the greatest intentions of sticking to your healthy way of eating, but then the triple layer fudge cake for Aunt Millie's 90th birthday or a co-workers retirement will be brought out. You decide to turn it down. Soon, the barrage will hit from those less disciplined. "Uh, why don't you lighten up and ENJOY life? You're going to die anyway." Sound familiar? This is where knowing what your destination and inspiration is can help you to stay self-disciplined. Very few others, though, will be able to understand or relate to such tenacity or resolute behavior.

However, success will come down to many such instances in your life, where you are going to have to look out for number one, at least when it comes to your own health. This is an arena in which no one else can do it for you. Several years ago, I met a gentleman who wanted to improve his physical condition and health. He had a few pounds to lose and was experiencing back problems that were hindering his life. He got started on a training program and made some significant progress initially. A few months down the road, he felt his progress had slowed down quite a bit. When we discussed this, he stated that he was performing his exercise routine on a regular basis. I guessed that the problem was related to what he was eating. I asked the gentleman to complete a three-day food diary. A three-day food diary is when a person writes down everything they eat and drink for three days. The man did this, and for the most part, his food intake looked within acceptable standards. However, I notice that every night at about 8:00pm, he was having a small bowl of orange sherbet. Orange sherbet on a nightly basis is not part of the formula for success. When I asked the gentleman about this, he told me a little more about his struggle. He said that every night he got cravings, and a little battle went on in his mind. You know, the "should I or shouldn't I" fight between our ears. This man was losing the struggle. Virtually every night he gave into his cravings, and had his orange sherbet and thus was failing to reach his healthiness goals. I asked him, "What has that sherbet ever really done for you? Has the sherbet ever really made any positive difference in your life?" He pondered the point for a moment, smiled and said, "not really". Sherbet or any other obstacle, gives us the *momentary* **illusion** of comfort and satisfaction. But this momentary comfort does not last, *really* does not satisfy in the long run, and often keeps us from our best. It is my belief that when this man taps into an inspiration in his life that is *STRONGER* than his desire to satisfy a temporary taste bud craving, he will more often overcome the call of the sherbet. He might still give in on occasion, but that will happen less and less as he progresses towards what really matters to him.

Many people view self-discipline as a negative. They see it as self-deprivation, Spartan-like, and just not much "fun". Nothing could be further from the truth. Let's take a brief look at some of the benefits and characteristics those who become more self-disciplined enjoy. Those who learn to be self disciplined end up getting far *MORE* out of life than those who continue to give in to their weaker nature. More "goodies", so to speak, that makes a real, lasting and momentous contribution to life. Remember, unless you have an inspiration that is strong, a "higher calling" of some sort, you will probably continue to consistently "cave in" when it comes to self-discipline.

Benefits and Qualities of Self-Disciplined People

1) **Self-disciplined people develop strength of character.** Circumstances have less impact on those who are disciplined. They keep their eyes on the prize. They adapt to and respond to challenges. They keep working relentlessly, much like the tortoise in Aesop's fables. Self discipline has been described as, "doing what you should do, when you should do it, whether you feel like it or not, and whether you want to or not". If you are going to attempt to live out the lifestyle depicted in this book, you can expect to face times when you don't *feel* like or *want* to exercise. If you persevere, despite those "feelings", you will develop strength of character that copes with adversity and takes advantage of opportunities as they come your way.

2) **They live in reality.** Self-disciplined people understand that life will never get "easy". Television commercials and advertising tell us, "we deserve a break today, etc., etc.". But the fact is, every day presents its challenges. There is only one place where there are no

problems, and that is six feet under. While there are times of rest, self-disciplined people understand that life is not meant to be a vacation 24-7. So many people live lives of futility because they are waiting for a life free of struggle; when they can just kick back and relax. Self-disciplined people have faced the fact that life is tough. At the same time, they realize it is full of adventure and an incredible opportunity. They are not sadists or Spartans because they enjoy being tough on themselves, but because they have learned, as Zig Ziglar says, "If you are first tough on yourself, life will be easier on you".

3) **They have less stress in their lives.** Because they have a system in place to continually improve all areas of their lives, they have *less* anxiety about the events and situations in their life. Granted, no one has total control over life. Tragedy, crisis, and accidents happen to all of us at some time or another. Because they have a plan for each of the significant areas of their life, self-disciplined people at least feel that they are in the front seat, rather than in the trunk, wondering what the heck is going to happen next. Health and fitness authorities agree that in times of increased stress, the best response is to actually increase exercise to combat the tearing down of the body and immune system that stress can cause. Self-disciplined people already have the stress reduction system in place before the stressor events occur.

4) **They operate out of faith/belief principles.** Abe Lincoln said, "I shall prepare myself, and someday, perhaps, my chance will come". He had faith that his day would dawn. The word faith is used in many ways in our culture, but its origin comes from the Bible where it is used to describe a trust in God. Faith is defined as, "hope in things that are unseen". Faith is similar to belief, and belief has more power than circumstances, talent, money, or anything else we can think of. This has been proven time after time after time through history. Those who are self-disciplined are employing this principle to improve their own lives. They continually put forth effort towards a positive goal, knowing that if they simply stay with it, eventually

it will pay off. Sometimes this must be done, even when there seems to be no evidence of anything getting better or changing. That is self-discipline in action. This is one of the biggest challenges facing people who attempt to take up a healthiness lifestyle, because they want to *see* results instantaneously. This dilemma has already been addressed, but if we can stay focused and self-disciplined, eventually we can achieve our objectives, sometimes to a greater degree than we ever dreamed. I have been physically training for thirty years now, and I continue to make improvements year after year, month after month, day after day, sometimes without me being aware of the improvements that incrementally occur. I simply *believe* that good efforts, done consistently over time, will pay off in something good. It always has. This principle, of course, works in all areas of life. It is different than just "having faith" and then not doing anything. Rather, it is the belief and consistent action *in combination* that produces awesome results.

I am convinced that none of us will achieve the fitness success possible for us unless we have belief and effort working together continuously. Exactly how they work together I do not fully comprehend. But I (and many others) can state emphatically, they do. Sometimes the question comes up, which comes first, the chicken (effort) or the egg (belief). I would submit that in the case of fitness, belief comes first. For if a person believes that there is hope, they are more likely to implement effort in a positive progressive manner.

5) **They have *MORE* freedom in their lives.** Many people assume the opposite. They view self-disciplined people as living by a bunch of rules, burdens and boundaries. If one were to take a closer look, they would see that the opposite is true. Those who are lacking in self-discipline are usually burdened by their life circumstances far more than those who are self-disciplined. For example, most of those who are too un-disciplined to exercise have less energy, are less fit, and are therefore less optimistic about their future healthiness. The opposite is true of the disciplined. They have learned that by "subjecting" themselves to bouts of short tem effort,

they get to *enjoy* lengthier periods of long-term comfort. Whereas those who cling to brief periods of comfort often end up enduring agonizingly long periods of discomfort or the sufferings of poor health. Sorry to be so blunt, but that is the truth. Even in a country with all of the freedoms we enjoy and resources for fitness available to us, many are in pitiful bondage to poor or mediocre health because they resist the structure of discipline.

> *"In the last analysis, our only freedom is the freedom to discipline ourselves"*
>
> Bernard Baruch

IV. Imagin-ation.

> *"Everything you can imagine, is real."*
>
> Pablo Picasso

> *"Ideas ultimately govern behavior."*
>
> Warren Bennis

> *"As a man thinks in his heart, so is he."*
>
> Proverbs

In ancient times, the heart was synonymous with the mind. The proverb above warns us to be careful about what we let into our minds and what we allow ourselves to dwell on. The word imagination, when broken down, is the "image in" our heads. The image of ourselves that we hold in our heads influences our health to a great extent. Allow me to illustrate. A few months back, a personal trainer contacted me with a question. She could not understand why some clients start training with her, got excited about making positive changes, began making significant progress, and then suddenly dropped out of sight. Several months later, she would run into them at the grocery store only to find that they had either returned to their previous condition, or in fact, worsened. She wanted to know why I thought this happened? I told her that I have come to believe that the image we have of ourselves, functions as a magnet in our lives. It determines what we are attracted to and what we avoid. I do not mean for this to be some self-help, pop psychology fodder. The fact is, what we think determines who we are and who we eventually become. Henry Ford said, "Whether we think (imagine) we can or think (imagine) we can't, we are probably right."

For example, a person may start a new fitness program, and have some success for a period of time. But if their self-image, (who they **imagine** themselves to be), remains unchanged, the gravitational pull of their self-limiting beliefs will always pull them back to their old, familiar, and less productive ways of functioning. And while those ways may not be healthy and could even be harmful, they *are* more comfortable. Lasting change requires a change in self-image. To many, this process seems scary, too risky, or they simply do not know where to begin. But the fact remains, the way we "imagine" ourselves will be the driving force and final determinant of our long-term results.

It is very difficult for people to consistently act beyond who and what they believe themselves to be. It is my guess that my friend's clients *imagine* themselves to be lazy, low-energy, or perhaps non-athletic, etc, people. Deep down inside, they can't truly see themselves as making permanent, successful changes in their lifestyle. Perhaps they can't see themselves as being able to turn back the clock, loose *all* the weight, undo the damage, exercise daily and like it, eat differently *forever*, etc. They can try a new lifestyle for a season but eventually; the call of the familiar takes over and takes control. They end up going back to their old, comfortable ways because the healthier version of life, "just isn't them". Or so they imagine.

According to Zig Ziglar, the "imagination is the strongest *nation* in the world". *Everything* starts there. In the case of imagination versus will power, imagination will always win. Let's say you decide to "get in shape". You set your goals, hire a trainer, etc. You are excited about getting started. The morning of your first appointment comes. The alarm clock rings, and the thoughts start to do a little dance. Perhaps they go something like this: "Oh man. Is it time to get up already? I shouldn't have scheduled for the morning. I feel better later in the day when I have more energy". You know you should get up and go anyway and you *want* to, but . . . . you begin to imagine yourself sweating, experiencing a little discomfort. You say to yourself, "I really have so much I have to do today. I'll fit it in later. Besides if I work out now, I might not have enough energy to get through the rest of the day." You begin to imagine (think) about the money this gym or trainer is going to cost you, and how you would rather spend it on something else. You imagine how nice it would be to sleep a little longer and figure all this out later. And in those few short moments, your imagination scores a victory over your will power. Naturally, this scenario may not exactly describe your particular challenge or circumstance, but I am confident that most of you can relate to some of it, whether you are trying to quit smoking, drinking or eat better. In each and every area of our lives, imagination will *always* be stronger than will power in the long run. Imagination can play a role in taking us to defeat, or be trained to take us to victory.

So what is the answer? How can we utilize the imagination for our future benefit? Scripture tell us that we should, "cast down all imaginations" that are not helpful. Assertive, almost aggressive action is necessary. First, negative imaginations (beliefs) must be identified. As a fitness trainer, I have found that one of the best ways to do this is by listening to people. Usually their conversations reveal who they truly *imagine* themselves to be. However, a problem for many is that they believe lies about themselves. Many believe they are not valuable, not meant to succeed, just average. For example, one woman I talked with described herself as a "sloth". Not surprisingly, she stated that exercising and being physically active have always been a struggle for her. Now, we cannot be sure which came first, but imagining or describing oneself as a sloth is certainly not helpful to becoming active and fit. Holding that image in ones mind would likely lead to moving and behaving like a sloth.

Another way to think of it is this. It has been said that, "like begets like". If you planted corn you would get corn, peas would get peas, etc. It is the same thing with the imagination. If you want to become fit and active, you must start "imaging" yourself as being that way. We are not talking about denying reality. If you are unfit, overweight, etc, then that is reality. But, if you hope to move beyond that, you must begin changing the images in your thinking. It's kind of like looking into the future, imagining a different way of life and choosing to believe in the coming reality of that image. If the woman who saw herself as a sloth, would start imagining herself as a cheetah (sticking with the animal theme), that would certainly begin to impact her behavior. This may sound a little "out there" but it works and is powerful. Many people have been negatively labeled or label themselves in regards to their physical appearance or abilities. A first step, then, would be to start listening to your self. What have you imagined or labeled yourself to be? Pay attention to that, because it WILL determine where you arrive.

I would like to share a simple "roadmap to results" that might help you to better understand why it is so important to be aware of how we think about ourselves. I learned of this straightforward idea a few years ago, and it has helped me to improve my life in several areas.

It goes like this:

- **Thinking** (imagination) leads to our
- **Beliefs** lead to our
- **Expectations** lead to our
- **Attitudes** lead to our
- **Actions** (or lack of) ultimately creating our
- **Results** (or lack of)

This roadmap holds true for every area of our lives. I have seen it in action time and again. With this roadmap in mind, a goal is to strive not to think or say anything to yourself that you **do not want** to result in your life.

Begin by thinking about how you currently imagine yourself in a physical sense. Is it positive and motivating, or more of a putdown that demoralizes and causes you to feel like a failure? A friend of mine recently told me that his weight has been, "a lifelong struggle. This has always been a problem for me". While that may be true, I think that a big part of his problem is how he talks to himself. He *thinks* (imagines) this is such a struggle, so he *believes* it will be a struggle, *expects* it to be a struggle leading to a defeated *attitude* that causes him not to try (no *action*) or to try half-hearted. In the end, he will get poor *results*. For many, what I just described has been a vicious, never ending cycle of defeat, which unfortunately has gone on for a lifetime. For change to take place, one must usually "hit bottom" and become seriously sick and tired of being sick and tired. Begin by *planting* new thoughts in your imagination. My friend would be well served to begin by saying something like, "I am **looking forward** to becoming leaner, healthier, and stronger. I have the information and tools to do it. I want to do it and I will do it, come heck or high water". If he continues to plant seeds *favorable* to fitness into his imagination, while pulling out the weeds of his past defeated and discouraging images, he will have a far greater chance of having a flourishing fitness future.

V. Deline-ation.

> *"Goals that are not written down are just wishes."*
> *Anonymous*

> *"Every day you spend drifting away from your goals is a waste not only of that day, but also of the additional day it takes to regain lost ground."*
> *Anonymous*

"Goals are dreams with deadlines."
Diana Scharf Hunt

Imagining yourself as a leaner, healthier or stronger person is only half of the battle. The other half will require *acting* on that imagination. Action itself may be of little good unless it is intelligent, effective action. I have known and watched people who for years put forth action towards getting healthier, but with little or poor results. They would go to the gym and move casually between pieces of equipment, do a few sets here and there, and call it good. They would take a few weeks off now and then when "something came up". There approach was "willy-nilly" and the results were not impressive. Not surprisingly, they often end up frustrated or at the very least, stagnated. Much of their problem was that they never really decided *exactly* what they wanted to accomplish. The word delineate means, "to line out" or to put in writing. Do you have physical fitness and health goals? Are they written down somewhere? Are they specific, with action steps and dates for accomplishment? If you do not have a formula, a system, or a plan, it is highly likely that **YOU WILL FAIL.**

One of the first experiments in the use of written goals took place over fifty years ago. In 1953 researchers polled the graduating class of Yale University and found that only 3% of the graduates practiced goal setting and had a set of clearly defined WRITTEN goals.

In 1973 researchers went back and visited the class of '53 and found that the 3 % of the graduates who had the clear and written goals had amassed a fortune worth more than the other 97 % combined! This is powerful evidence that goal setting is a proven process for improving any area of our lives. Since that time, many other successful people have used the principle of specific written goals to improve their results.

As I have traveled the country presenting at seminars, I sometimes ask who in the audience has specific written goals for their life. Surprisingly, only about 3-5 % of the audience raises their hands. Experts tell us the reason goal setting is so effective is that it "turns on" our reticular activating system (RAS). The RAS is thought to be a part of the brain that acts like a heat seeking missile and leads us to information, people and opportunities in line with our goal. The more specific the goal, the better our brain can help us, and when we write it down, it is almost like "imprinting" it onto our brain. Whether or not this is truly *how* it works is up for debate, yet I can state with absolute certainty that this *does* work. And, if you are serious about wanting exceptional health, fitness and wellness results, writing down your goals is the first step. This benefits and improves our lives by:

> Giving us direction and energy.
> Organizing our thoughts and time.
> Adjusting our attitudes to ones of optimism and hope.
> Learning self discipline.
> Seeing our significance and enhanced capacity to serve others
> by improving ourselves.

In conversations with people regarding written goal setting, I have heard the f-word more times than I can count. That's right, FEAR. Sometimes minor fear; sometimes deep, debilitating fears keep people in bondage. This is a very real issue that must be addressed. Fear is monumental in the lives of many and beyond the scope of this book. But this much I know, one of the best ways to start erasing and defeating a fear or any other obstacle, is by having an action plan to reduce them while increasing what we need more of in our lives. Henry Ford said it well; "Obstacles are those frightful things you see when you take your eyes off your goal". Accordingly, you must first have a goal. But the thought of actually writing out a fitness goal often ends up exposing our hidden fears.

So before we discuss how to write a goal, lets take a brief look at some of the fears that people have in regards to taking up an improved lifestyle of healthiness. Some of the fears and concerns individuals admit include the following:

- Fear of hurting oneself or getting injured
- Fear of being uncomfortable
- Fear of looking/feeling awkward
- Fear of failing
- Fear of change

Take note that at least four of these fears are *MORE* likely to happen without a written goal and action plan to make things better. For instance, people are *already* literally "falling apart" from not taking action to improve their physical condition and are suffering from a greater degree of debilitating diseases and ailments. They are *already* in the process of **hurting and injuring** themselves by idly sitting. Passivity leads to being uncomfortable. The person experiences failure by default in their physical condition. Changes—negative ones— will follow including lack of mobility, difficulty working hard, illness, stiff joints, inability to enjoy previous activities, the list goes on.

Naturally, when attempting something new, many people fear looking or feeling awkward. I know people who have expressed that they are not athletic. They lack confidence that they will be able to succeed in exercising. If this is a fear for you, realize this: everyone is an athlete, some just naturally posses more ability than others. Getting out of a chair is an athletic event most of us do everyday. Walking requires coordination. Like these activities, others that you will learn will ultimately happen smoothly and with little thought.

At first, some of these movements may indeed feel awkward and it will take your body, nerves, and muscles a little while to adjust. But exercising is a skill, much like casting a fishing pole, swinging a golf club, or whipping an egg. You must push through the awkward learning phase to enjoy the benefits. Trust me, *ANYONE* can do the exercises found in this book. Ninety year olds who needed a walker to get around have been successful. So can you. Write out what success would be for you and write out an action plan to get it done. As you do, your body will turn into one that has less hurts and less *chance* of getting hurt. You will learn little by little to take your body to reasonable momentary stints of mild discomfort, in order to realize the benefits of long-term feelings of true comfort and confidence. You will begin to feel more and more successful.

By the way, for now, consider yourself successful if you simply put your goals in writing and then complete three workouts per week. The mass media would tell us that success is looking like Sally or Sam supermodel. Don't buy the lie. If you can write out your goals and then follow through with three workouts per week, you will be more successful than 90% of the population in this country.

Still hesitant? What if you approached the other important parts of your life with no game plan? If you want no results or poor results, avoid this issue of goal setting. Otherwise, write your goals on the form at the end of this section. Hear me now, believe me later . . . it certainly can't hurt to try.

THERE IS GOLD IN GOALS!
"I am a slow walker, but I don't walk backwards".
Abraham Lincoln

"You may be disappointed if you fail, but you are doomed if
you don't try".
Beverly Sills

The power of goal setting is undeniable. Only a very small percentage of people in the world have **written specific goals** and they outperform all others in similar endeavors. They virtually leave others in the dust. Putting your goals, dreams, or vision in writing is a step of faith. Let's begin by thinking about and answering the following questions. These aren't your goals, but considering these questions will help you design the right goals for you.

1. **How would you like to see yourself health, fitness and wellness in six months?** Be realistic, but don't be afraid to dream. Be as specific as possible and frame it in the positive. For example: I would like to weigh a lean, fit, and strong 190 lbs, able to perform 25 pushups and run a mile in under 8 minutes. This is better than saying, "I want to lose weight and get in better shape".

    _____

    _____

    _____

2. **Where are you now in relation to that goal??** Put it in writing. For example, I currently weigh 235 lbs, can do 2 pushups, and jog a ½ mile in 8 minutes.

    _____

    _____

3. **Why is the goal important to you?**

    _____

    _____

4. **What will happen if you don't do this?**

    _____

    _____

5. **What could happen and what would it be like if you achieved this goal?**

    _____

    _____

6. **What fears might you have about attempting this goal?**

    _____

    _____

7. How could you overcome these fears?

_____

_____

8. What obstacles/challenges will you face?

_____

_____

9. How can you overcome these obstacles?

_____

_____

9) What action steps are needed on your part to accomplish this goal?

_____

_____

10) What reasons and excuses are you using or are you likely to encounter that will prevent you from getting started today or tonight?)

_____

_____

Now that you have thought about or answered those questions, it is time to write your own clear and concise written fitness goal. The objective is to have your goal, along with action steps, written on a 3 x 5 index card.

So how do we write a goal to improve our fitness, health, and wellness? Many goal-writing experts suggest that your goals be S. M. A. R. T. That is, they should be specific, measurable, achievable, realistic, and with timelines. This goal setting "formula" has been around for years, and with good reason. Goals that have a specific, measurable target with a deadline have a much better chance of being accomplished. Where many people get off track are in the "achievable and realistic" areas. An achievable goal should be one that can be broken down into doable steps. For instance, if your goal is to run a

24-mile marathon and you have never run before, you would not start off by trying to run 24 miles. Instead, you would likely start with one mile and progressively build your distance. Realistic means what it says. If you are five foot tall, 55 years old and 300 pounds, setting a goal to be able to dunk a basketball might not be realistic. Instead, setting a goal to increase your vertical jump by 2 inches might be a more sensible and doable goal.

It is a good idea to consider the S.M.A.R.T. formula above when designing your goal. In addition, because our goals in this case involve our physical fitness, I like to recommend that you take into account four aspects in your written health goal. Some of these components were mentioned in the above questions. These are; how you want to improve **physically**, how you want to improve **performance-wise**, why this goal is **important** to you, and **when** you want to accomplish this by (date). This is your goal *statement,* and will be written on one side of a 3 x 5 index card. For example, a recent client came to me weighing in at 270 pounds, and unable to jog for more than three minutes. He was also on three medications.

His goal stated, "that he wanted to weigh 190 lean, strong and fit pounds, (The physical improvement), and be able to jog one mile and able to perform 25 pushups, (The performance improvement), in order to get off all three medications and be around to see his grandchildren grow up (Importance). He set a goal to do this within six months (When). All of that fit neatly on the front of the card.

On the reverse side of the card he wrote the following action steps:

1) I will weight train three days per week, thirty minutes per day every Mon-Wed-Fri. I will always be on time for my workouts, and will call ahead if for any reason I might be late.

2) On my non-weight training days I will ride a recumbent bicycle for 20 minutes at the correct intensity level or walk briskly uphill for 20 minutes. I will do this on Sat-Tues-Thurs, and take Sundays off.

3) I will write down *everything* I eat and drink *every* day, following the guidelines I have been instructed in. I will turn in my written food diaries once per week for evaluation.

4) I will eat an average of six meals per day, every 2.5-3.5 hours. Breakfast will be eaten within 15-20 minutes of waking up.

5) I will only eat junk food once per week, on Friday nights.

He kept a copy of this, and so did I. His results were remarkable. You can do the same. Write out your goal on a 3-x5 card with action steps. Give a copy to a trusted encourager in your life. Read the card once a week, *follow the action steps* and chances are good you will enjoy many new improvements this year, and for years to come.

It should look something like this.

My Goal
Statement _____
_____
_____

Action Step I.
_____
_____

Date to accomplish _____

Action Step II.
_____
_____

Date to accomplish _____

Action Step III.
_____
_____

Date to accomplish _____

Action Step III.
_____
_____

Date to accomplish _____

Action Step V.
_____
_____

Date to accomplish _____

My Signature _____
My accountability partner/coach signature _____
Dated

VI. Habitu-ation.

"Habit is a shirt made of Iron."

Anonymous

"Old habits are strong and jealous."

Dorthea Brande

"Habit is the deepest law of human nature."

Thomas Carlyle

Initiation, destination, inspiration, imagination, and delineation, though powerful in our lives, are still not enough. For anything to become a permanent part of our lives, it must become a habit. The good news is that all of us are already using habits in our lives. Virtually everything that we think and do is habit. The bad news is that the habits we have are not always helping us. For example, 90 out of 100 Americans are in the habit of not getting enough physical exercise to receive **any** fitness benefits. Sixty out of one hundred Americans are considered sedentary. The good news is that this is something we can change. Three things are needed if we don't want to be part of the unfit majority. First, we need to define a habit. Second, we need an understanding of the process by which habits work in our lives. Finally, we need to know how to remove bad habits and replace them with good ones.

Habituation means, "to bring into a condition or habit of the body". The definition of a habit is, "something done often and hence, easily". I would add that these things are usually done without thinking. As a result, we sometimes continue doing them without regard to their consequence, whether or not they are really of benefit to our lives in the long term.

Some habits are described as addictive, such as smoking. Because of the chemical effects of nicotine, we become physically hooked, and it is very tough to "kick the habit". I submit to you, however, that *all* habits are actually addictive. That is why they have become a habit. They temporarily make us feel comfortable, give us pleasure, or make us feel safe. Perhaps they do all three.

The problem is that some of our habits are not healthy and some control us, rather than we controlling them. Either way, habits ultimately determine our fate, our future, and our destiny. If our habits are good, that is good news. But a review of popular Americans health habits reveals that our habits are slowly but surely squeezing the life out of us. How do we undo poor habits and replace them with rich, rewarding and productive ones? First, let's take a look at how they start in the first place.

We earlier reviewed the importance of imagination in our lives. Imagination is simply a form of thinking which is the starting point for all habits. It goes something like this:

> *Think a thought (imagination) often enough, and eventually you will grow an action (which could mean to do nothing). That action or lack of, done often enough becomes a habit. That habit done often enough becomes our character and that character then has control over our lives and our destiny. This is why it is so critical to evaluate what we think about. Our thinking is where it all starts. We can unravel the bad habits that may be holding back or hurting our lives, by first becoming aware of and then changing the way we think.*

Let me explain how to do this by giving you a visual image of how habits work in our lives. Habits operate as steel cables in our daily living. As you may know, steel cables are incredibly strong, virtually impossible to break or even cut in half. Steel cables, however, are made up of hundreds of tiny steel cables, all wound together. By themselves, each cable, while durable, could easily be snipped. It is the same thing with habits. Each time we have performed or failed to perform a behavior, it is like a single strand of a steel cable. Repeated over time, we have built the behavior into a steel cable **habit**, that all of the forces of will power in the world could not overcome. However, by slowly, and progressively peeling away one strand of the habit each day, and purposefully replacing that strand with a better habit strand, we can build new cables into our lives, which can hoist us to new heights of healthiness.

To illustrate: If you have been an inactive "couch potato" for the past twenty years, you now have a lot of tiny steel cables of inactivity built into your life. You must develop a plan to remove them a little each day over the next weeks, months, years and decades. At the same time, replace those habits with behaviors such as the ones outlined in this book. I realize this may sound like tedious work, much slower than all of the overnight solutions you are sold on late night TV. You and I know, however, that this is the ultimate fitness and health truth. And, the truth is, it really doesn't take *that* long to get results. It is the only thing that works for a lifetime, and it is worth it.

Several years ago, I was training a gentleman named Jack. Jack was in his early seventies and was recovering from a stroke. He started off on his training with vigor and enthusiasm. For the first few weeks, he showed up for his workouts early, raring to go. After about three weeks though, he began to lose steam. Finally one day, I inquired as to the reasons for his change of heart. Jack responded, "well I'm really enjoying some of the results I am getting and I'm feeling much better. But I am actually a bit disappointed as well". I asked him the cause of his disappointment and he responded, "My belly". "What about your belly?" I asked. "Well Fred, I still have it", he noted patting the pillow that existed in place of his waistline. "Yes Jack?" I mused. "Well, I thought it would be gone by now", he said. Knowing that Jack was an intelligent man, I asked Jack how long it took him to get his belly? He thought for a moment and then responded, "About thirty five years". It didn't take Jack long to figure out that if it took him thirty five years to build that belly, it wasn't realistic to expect it to disappear in three weeks. I went on to explain that his quest for fitness was bigger than his belly. It was about his whole life. We agreed to focus on a healthy lifestyle and to let the belly take care of itself. That was ten years ago. Last time I saw Jack, his belly was far more refined and he was still actively enjoying his workouts. It is all about habit.

One last thought on this topic. Habits turn into routines, and routines, if we are not careful, can turn into ruts. A routine is all of our habits wrapped together into our day. We have different habits in each area of our lives, and we follow them day after day. This can be good.

Here are some thoughts about my daily routine: I prefer to call it a rhythm, as that sounds a little livelier and denotes a bit of flexibility. I spend time each day pursuing spiritual, intellectual, social, emotional and physical fitness interests. This helps me to stay balanced. Many experts in physical and mental health suggest a similar "routine". Routines/rhythms are one of the most positive tools available in reducing or minimizing stress in our lives. Many people do not use this idea, but instead approach their lives with a "go with the flow" approach. While flexibility is good and being a free spirit has its moments, a go with the flow lifestyle can sometimes cause us undue stress. We run the risk of being carried away by the flow, sometimes in a direction we don't want or like. We may find that we end up being swept by the "flow" into a sea of someone else's stress. Develop a routine or rhythm. Include fitness. Live life on purpose. Adapt your own rhythm. Health experts agree, that the more stress we have in our lives, the more we NEED to exercise and eat well. Write out your own rhythm today. Mine is given as an example.

Fred's RHYTHM/ROUTINE PLANNER Example

Wake and Eat: 5 a.m.

Read Bible & Study for
School: 5:30-6:30 a.m.

Workout: 6:30-7:00 a.m.

Ready for Work:
7:00-7:45 a.m.

Arrive at Work: 8:00 a.m.

Snack/Brunch: around 8 a.m.

Lunch: around 11:00 a.m.

Mid-Day Snack:—
around 2:00 p.m.

Leave Work: 5:00 p.m.

Dinner: 5:30 p.m.

Time with Family/Friends

Mid-Evening snack:
around 8:30 p.m.

Go to Sleep:
9:30/10:00 p.m.

Write out a daily "rhythm" for yourself. It does not have to be perfect the first time, but should include 15-30 minutes per day work toward your written health goals.

VII. Appreci-ation.

> *"Next to excellence is appreciation of it."*
> *William Makepeace Thackeray*

> *"We act as though comfort and luxury were the chief requirements of life, when all that we need to make us happy is something to be enthusiastic about."*
> *Charles Kingsley*

> *"Optimism is the faith that leads to achievement. Nothing can be done without hope and confidence."*
> *Helen Keller*

Appreciation is defined as, "to think well of" and to, "recognize gratefully". We have such a strong tendency to take things in life for granted, including our bodies. Often, it is not until they begin to fail us that we give them the care and attention that they require.

It seems fair to say that the majority of people view taking care of themselves as a burden. Exercising is so often described as a drag or chore and people often whine about having to watch what they eat. At the same time, many seem to wonder why they feel so lethargic. If they approached all of their life with such a disparaging attitude, the implications might not be pretty. But such is not the case. On the golf course or in the shopping mall their attitude is altogether different. They become almost, "light on their feet" with an unstoppable attitude of adventurous anticipation of what lies ahead.

If they could intentionally shift some of that seize-the-day attitude over to their fitness pursuits, they might find they begin to enjoy themselves. I know what I am describing seems unrealistic to many. But the fact is, if we can still walk and breath, we have much to appreciate, and to be grateful for. Many others have gone before us and many are currently risking their life and limb so that you and I can live and enjoy freedom and the pursuit of happiness and healthiness.

However, many of us are not making the best of what we have been given in the physical arena. On the whole, we are experiencing substandard levels of fitness and health. A major contributor to this predicament is our attitude towards a fitness lifestyle. Let's turn the tide of tired attitudes and make the most of what we've got, and fulfill our destiny in this one time shot. Lets begin to more fully appreciate what we've been given, to set an example for our young people of fully alive living. There are two attitudinal components of appreciation that we can look to, to take us to the finish line of success.

The first is optimism. Optimism has been defined as, "the tendency to take the most hopeful view of matters" and the, "belief that good ultimately prevails over bad". The opposite of optimism is of course, pessimism. Pessimism is the, "tendency to always expect the worst", and that, "the bad in life outweighs the good". We all know people who tend to be optimists, and those who tend to be pessimists. Either quality taken to an extreme can be weird and difficult to endure for any length of time. But, of the two, a degree of realistic optimism is far more effective in having success in the pursuit of greater health and fitness. Optimism, in the case of exercising for example, is an undeterred belief that such activity is and will continue to provide real, measurable, and valuable results to every area of an individual's life, now and throughout their lives. This attitude usually produces what it expects.

Not only that, but there is credible evidence that optimists live longer and have a higher quality of life overall. For those of you who tend to be pessimistic, I would like to offer a word of encouragement. You need not convert to the ever-smiling Pollyanna, predictor of a brighter future, to make improvements here. Experts suggest that it is important that the pessimist not be **consumed** by negativity. Don't become a hard-hearted cynic, with a "life stinks and then you die" dogma as your personal motto. Pessimism isn't always a bad thing. We've all benefited from the healthy skepticism (which is sometimes lacking in overblown optimists) of the pessimist at some time. Skepticism can lead to a quest for more detail, more facts, and more review. That can sometimes save us from taking unproductive or even harmful action.

The key, according to researchers, is for those who tend to be pessimistic to simply become *less* pessimistic. It is simply a matter of not staying stuck in chronic defeated negativity that matters. Likewise, obsessively optimistic individuals can sometimes go too far with their, "life is terrific" attitude when the facts are spelling otherwise. Sometimes facing the facts is needed before we can start getting somewhere. Smiling all day may be better than a constant frown, but it may not improve your body fat percentage without a reality check and subsequent action to improve it.

It seems intelligent to face the facts of our current condition, and then optimistically take action to improve it. With that in mind, I'd like to outline 12 traits of balanced and effective optimists. These are from the exceptionally good book "*The Power of Optimism*", by Alan Loy McGinnis. Some of these traits do not directly apply to improving our fitness levels, but they all apply to improving the condition of our mind and emotions, which directly impacts health and wellness

- **Optimists are seldom surprised by trouble.** They see themselves as problem-solvers.
- **Optimists look for partial solutions.** Beginning is half the doing and they are people of action.
- **Optimists believe they have a degree of control over their future.** They are confident, and don't think other people's opinions should determine their reality.
- **Optimists allow time for regular renewal.** Exercising is seen as an opportunity to renew the physical, mental, emotional and spiritual self, not as a boring or burdensome event.
- **Optimists interrupt their negative trains of thought.** They monitor and question "automatic thoughts". Then, they actively and assertively replace distorted or false thoughts with ones of truth and progression.
- **Optimists heighten their power of appreciation.** They have already imagined what it would be like to lose their "blessings" so they are better able to savor what they currently possess.
- **Optimists use their imagination to rehearse success.** Pessimists use their imagination, but tend to do so with negative consequences in mind. Optimists, tend to imagine being successful, but are not disheartened or permanently defeated if things don't work out at the first few attempts.
- **Optimists are cheerful, even when they can't be happy.** Optimists are often committed exercisers. Even when things are not going well in their lives, they maintain this habit as an antidote to depression. They also tend to participate in spiritual calisthenics when the challenges of life seem overwhelming, such as reciting favorite scriptures: e.g . . . "This is the day . . ."
- **Optimists think they have great capacity for stretching.** Deep down inside, they firmly feel that the best is yet to come, that they have not yet reached their peak. They feel as Browning said, "Come grow old with me. The best is yet to be!"

- **Optimists build lots of love into their lives.** They work harder to understand others, giving people the benefit of the doubt. This keeps bitterness and resentment from strangling their spirit, and keeps the oxygen of encouragement flowing. They also tend to give more easily, from the perspective of, "I had no shoes and complained until I met a man with no feet".
- **Optimists like to swap good news.** They have an eye out for goodness accompanied by a desire to learn from what they see. They seek to incorporate similar meaningful and positive behaviors and qualities into their own lives and the lives of those they influence.
- **Optimists practice accepting what they cannot change.** Most unhappiness is a result of wanting something we don't have. Optimists question, "how can I make things better?" They tend to focus on what they can improve and let go of what they can't change/control

Some of the above traits may seem to have little to do with fitness. But if it is true that optimists live longer and have higher quality lives, wouldn't it be wise for us to consider how these twelve points impact our fitness endeavors?

Another area of attitude that separates those who stay stuck in the quagmire of mediocre health versus those who soar to new heights of healthiness is the quality of enthusiasm. Enthusiasm is taken from the Latin root, "Entheos", and means, "one who moves with the energy of the divine". It had its origins in the days of the early church, when the governing authorities were concerned about the religious "fanatics" who were displaying unbridled amounts of cheerful energy, which heretofore had been unseen, except in the case of those who consumed large amounts of wine. The current use of the word "fan", as it relates to sports, etc, is a shortening of the original, "fanatic". The enthusiasm of these early church members was seen as a danger. The governing authorities did not understand the origin of the enthusiasm and were afraid of losing control of the "fanatical" masses.

It is true that enthusiasm, used for the wrong purposes, can be destructive and even deadly. Hitler was certainly enthusiastic in his desire to rule the world. But enthusiasm was meant to produce good, not evil. Its power and effectiveness is undeniable. And, if you truly want to get great results, you would be remiss to dismiss its use in pursuing health and fitness. We have been hearing for years now about the obesity epidemic. Wouldn't it be great if instead we had an epidemic of enthusiasm and action in pursuing a fully alive lifestyle? While the chances of that happening aren't favorable, perhaps it would be plausible if we got a different perspective. Attitude, when you boil it all down, is really not a whole lot more than our perspective.

Several years ago I received a phone call from a woman named Dee-Dee who had been referred by a friend. It turns out that Dee-Dee had been to see her doctor and he was concerned about her health. He was especially concerned about her risk for diabetes and the high level of her blood pressure. We had a brief conversation and then we discussed her exercise habits. Dee-Dee informed me that this was a problem for her as she "hated to exercise". I then asked her what she did like and her answer was concise: "comfort". I explained to her that by exercising, she could actually *increase* the comfort in her life. But if she persisted in avoiding it, she might actually increase the amount of discomfort, suffering and inconvenience. We spent a few more moments discussing the benefits of exercise, and I sensed that I would probably lose her as a client, as this whole exercise idea was not what she had hoped to hear. Having nothing to loose, I decided to take a bit of a risk. I boldly suggested that she needed to change her attitude and become more enthusiastic about exercising. "Look Fred", she commented, "I will *never* become enthusiastic about exercising!" I went on to say that as long as she maintained a negative attitude, she could expect to feel negative. I also warned her that she would likely get average to poor results with the current level of enthusiasm she possessed.

On the other hand, I explained to her that if she became enthusiastic, she would find the drudgery feelings gradually give way to enjoyment and confidence. I reminded her that experts say enthusiasm towards a positive goal helps to strengthen our mental, emotional, and spiritual health. But she still wasn't buying it. Finally, in one last effort, I asked her if she was familiar with Christopher Reeves, the actor who had suffered a paralyzing accident and was now a quadriplegic. She assured me that she knew who he was. I asked Dee-Dee how she thought Christopher Reeves would feel if he had the opportunity to exercise. Can you imagine, I asked, if the doctors came to Christopher and said, "Chris, we've found a way for you to walk again. But, there is a catch. For the rest of your life, three days a week, you are going to have to exercise for 25-35 minutes. You will have to keep up the routine for as long as you desire to be able to walk and use your arms."

I asked Dee-Dee what she thought Christopher would say, and how he might feel. "Do you think that he would whine, and say, 'exercise, are you kidding, I hate to exercise, it's so boring, what a drag!' Or, do you think he would be enthusiastic? My guess is that he would pour forth tears of joy at the opportunity to exercise and move and take care of his body and his muscles. I bet his enthusiasm would be overwhelming and unstoppable." She agreed. "Dee-Dee", I said, "You and I have that opportunity today." At that, she soon hung up the phone. I thought for sure that I would never hear from her again. Much to my surprise, a few weeks later she called back. "I am *so* ready to get started!" she **ENTHUSIASTICALLY** declared. "I've got a new workout suit, new tennis shoes, and a new attitude", she added. "I'm curious, Dee-Dee, what has happened to you? Your outlook seems to have taken a turn for the better", was my response. She told me that after our conversation, and thinking it through, her perspective on taking care of her body had begun to change. According to her, she began to see that exercising, or the ability to do so, was actually a privilege, and something she had not *appreciated* before. And, I am pleased to testify that the last time I checked Dee-Dee was still exercising, and in hot pursuit of healthiness.

Optimism and enthusiasm are powerful assets to our lives, and I would submit *indispensable* keys to a fitness lifestyle. Depression is running rampant in America, yet many people are running *from* fitness. Incidentally, research has shown that three exercise sessions per week has the same effect as taking Zoloft (an anti-depressant). I would argue that exercise is a far better, cheaper, and healthier solution. New research is also indicating that many anti-depressants actually *increase* depression long term, sometimes even resulting in suicide.

At the same time that depression is burgeoning, boredom seems to be blossoming. Many of us waste valuable minutes and hours watching unproductive fantasy "reality" shows or the like. We could be using that time to discover and build our own enthusiastic and optimistic futures. People often say that they like to relax by watching TV, and then state that exercise is boring and not entertaining. The truth is, though, that it is our attitudes toward exercise that are boring. Yes, sometimes we have to get creative to make our exercise and fitness pursuits more interesting and enjoyable, but our perspective and mind-set is really the key. We can usually make any endeavor either more miserable or enjoyable, simply by the mental approach we decide to take. Let's work towards developing more optimism, enthusiasm, and appreciation towards the privilege we have to exercise and take care of our bodies.

VIII. Perspir-ation.

> *"Sweat is the cologne of accomplishment"*
> Unknown

> *"Mediocrity is climbing molehills without sweating"*
> Icelandic proverb

The Russians have long been revered for their superiority in physical training, health and athletics. One of their most basic, age-old prescriptions for good health is to break a sweat everyday.

The theory behind this is that it actually cleanses and purifies the body. For those of us who habitually and intentionally cause ourselves to sweat, I think you would agree that there is just something very refreshing about a good sweat. It obviously cleans the pores of the skin, but it also helps to improve blood circulation. I am sure that there are other health benefits as well, but the bottom line is, if we are sweating, we have likely been exerting ourselves, which we KNOW produces many benefits in our lives.

In conversations with those who do not like to sweat (usually the ladies), I have heard comments like, "it just feels icky, it's not very feminine, or the infamous, "then I'd have to change my clothes". I suppose these concerns might have a smidgen of validity, but let's get serious. "Icky" is being unhealthy, diseased, and exhausted. Furthermore, not having the correct amount of muscle on your skeleton, while carrying an excess of body fat is not all that pleasant either. It limits your life and your ability to participate in activities. You can buy more clothes, but you really can't buy a new body. Yes, it has been said that America is becoming a "Frankenstein" nation with all of the plastic surgeries, but the fact is that we can never replace our muscles, bones, hearts, etc. with anything *nearly* as good as what we were originally given.

I think its safe to say that most men find a woman that takes care of herself—even though it involves sweating—more appealing than one who doesn't put forth the effort to fine tune what she has been given. By the same token, many women I speak to at conferences have said that they wish their husbands would take better care of themselves. Each of us will survive a little perspiration. Most of us will thrive better if we make it a goal to purposefully bring about a sweat, at least three days a week, by forcing our muscles to do a little bit more than they are used to do doing in a focused exercise session.

People who avoid perspiring like the plague are usually the ones plagued by ongoing illness, disease and/or substandard health. They avoid the perceived misery of exerting themselves, meanwhile enduring the very real misery of agonizing operations, body impairing medications and life threatening ailments. This makes no sense, yet it's without a doubt the futile experience of millions. Those who have learned to progressively push their bodies to the point of perspiring, get to "glisten" in the glow of growing strength, vitality and health. Unfortunately, however, many of us have to learn these things the hard way.

Several years' back, I worked with a woman who was always asking me health and fitness questions. She was interested in shedding a few extra pounds of body fat, and improving her health and energy levels. I gave her some of my handouts to read, and she returned them to me, and stated that, "it looks interesting, but it looks like too much work. Show me something I can do where I don't have to sweat!". Her solution, she informed me, was to buy a treadmill. I told her, that a treadmill could provide a little benefit, but compared to other options, using *solely* a treadmill was like going to a gourmet banquet of foods, and eating the crumbs off the floor. Perhaps a bit of an exaggeration I will admit, but I wanted her to get the message. I told her that treadmills were the most commonly purchased piece of home fitness equipment, and the results seem to speak for themselves. Our nations health and fitness is not getting better, it's getting worse. I suggested that if the treadmill were actually going to help her, it would only do so if she pushed herself to the point of sweating a little while using it.

Over the years I have learned that the adage, a person convinced against their will, is of the same opinion still" holds true in most cases. So, I shut my mouth, and waited to hear the tale of this woman's progress. She would occasionally touch base, and complain that things weren't really getting any better. Then, unfortunately, she fell and broke her leg while walking on the beach. The fall literally shattered her leg, and she was forced to miss several months of work. Eventually she did return but she was hobbling and hampered by her condition. She also continued to experience chronic pain. Finally, one day while passing by her in the hall, she stopped me. "Fred, she said, what can I do? I have gone to physical therapy, the doctors have done all that they can, and they tell me it will just take time. But it has been months, and things are not getting any better. The pain is almost unbearable." She began to get tears in her eyes as she described this agony. I paused for a moment, and responded, "First off, I am not a doctor. But this much I know. I have given you the best information available on the planet to take the average human body to its absolute best operating and performing condition. Up to this point, you haven't taken advantage of it. I am convinced that you will not get completely better, until you stop relying on others to give you an easy solution. No doctor, physical therapist, chiropractor or even personal trainer will be able to do this for you. You are going to have to decide to do the work (i.e. sweat). Until then, you will not really get much better."

Now, that may sound harsh, but realize that we had known each other for years and I felt that she trusted me. Still, I was concerned that I might have discouraged or offended her. Her birthday came up a few weeks later, and I gave her a copy of the book, *Strong Women Stay Young*. (My book was not done yet!). In the weeks that followed, we didn't discuss fitness. However, I began to notice that her clothes were beginning to look a little baggy. Finally, one day she stopped into my office and said, "Okay, you were right. The treadmill was play compared to this weight lifting stuff. My muscles were sore at first from even tiny weights. I'm starting to increase my weight amounts though and I feel *so* much better. Thank you for your willingness to take a hard line with me."

I could be wrong of course, but I can't help but think that if she had taken up this lifestyle previous to her fall, she may have avoided falling in the first place; breaking any bones or perhaps the injury would not have been so severe. A few weeks later, while at a work function, I sat next to this woman and her husband. She said to me, "Fred, tell him. Tell him all the things you told me. He won't listen to me." It seems her husband had been diagnosed with a "heart condition" and his doctor had told him to avoid "strenuous" activity. I told him that I didn't know his doctor, but I would get a few more opinions, because that sounded like a prescription for limited living. He told me that my formula sounded like, "too much work".

We all make our choices. I hope you choose to start sweating more. You will feel less icky. Bring a change of clothes along with your changed attitude. Learn to start enjoying and benefiting from a "prescription" of perspiration.

IX. Restor-ation.

"So many people spend their health gaining wealth, and then have to spend their wealth regaining their health"
A.J. Reb Materi

An interesting principle has been learned in the study of centenarians. We discussed this a bit at the start of the book but I felt it needed to be touched on again here. Centenarians, as you may recall, are those individuals who have been able to live to at least 100 years of age. It turns out that those who live that long— while successfully maintaining their health, vigor and independence—possess a common thread. This thread is what has been labeled, "the hardiness factor". This factor represents the ability to handle difficulty, and while in the midst of it, stand strong. It is strength of mindset, emotion and resolve coupled with the wisdom to know when it's time to restore lost energy. Many of us have not wised up to this valuable practice. Instead, we live our lives at a frenetic pace, thinking that the world and everyone around us will fall apart if we don't get this and that done. And we don't know when to rest.

One of the practical ways that centenarians practice hardiness is by taking "time out" during the day to restore them selves. Regardless of the circumstances, stressors, or tragedies going on around them, they make it a priority to take a quick nap, sit down and relax, or rest their head on a desk for a few moments. Most centenarians also say that they spend time each day in brief, effective exercise sessions. This is another way of restoring themselves. By maintaining muscle strength and flexibility, they pull in oxygen to refresh the blood supply to the heart and lungs. They habitually do this regardless of what is going on in their lives at the time. They have learned, that in the midst of stress, heartbreak over loss, serious health issues etc., they must keep themselves "fortified" to handle the demands of life. Otherwise, they may find themselves succumbing to the negative effects of high-level stress and become unable to help care for others or maintain the high degree of functioning they enjoy. Follow their lead. Don't neglect your self physically, *even* during times of high stress and problems. As has been said throughout this book, during periods of exceptionally high stress, we actually need to *increase* exercise and activity.

A few years back, the sales manager of a national company regularly came to my office to take our weekly food order. This guy was one of the most decent, professional people I have ever had the pleasure to do business with. We usually had light-hearted conversations about sports and current events. Now and again, though, we would talk about the increasing stress he felt from the demands of his work. He would always say, "I've got to start doing something to deal with this stress". I shared my usual "lifestyle speech" to which he always responded, "you're right, I need to get started. And I will, as soon as things slow down. I have wanted to do something to get in shape, but life just seems to always get in the way. If it is not something at work, it seems like projects at home are staring me in the face". I suggested that things will likely *never* slow down and asked him about his health goals? He replied, "My goals are to lose about 50 pounds and to quit smoking". "Well, I responded, we could get started on that tomorrow if you want. Meet me at the gym tomorrow morning and we'll get started. We'll train three days per week (for free), for about 30-35 minutes, and you will be well on your way to reaching your goals". He then said the all too common, "let me think about it".

A few weeks later, *he* brought the topic up again. He said, "you know Fred, I have thought about what you said, and I think I'd like to wait on exercising until I quit smoking". I had heard excuses like this many times and I decided to be straight with him. I asked him, "How long do you want to live?" He thought for a moment, and then responded, "Eighty. Eighty would be good". I went on to ask, "What do you want the remaining years of your life to be like? Would you like them to be excellent, dynamic and alive, or mediocre, maligned and maybe even miserable?" He responded, of course with "excellent". He went on to say that he was 38 years old and felt awful. As clearly as I could, I let him know that I didn't think he would make it to 50 if he maintained his current lifestyle. He looked at me seriously and said, "I know, I know. But seriously, Fred, as soon as I quit smoking, I'll start training with you." I saw my friend many, many times after that day. We would occasionally touch on the topic of health and stress, but I knew that things wouldn't change until he was ready.

Unfortunately, he never got the chance. About five months after our serious conversation, I received a phone call, informing me that he had died at 39 years old from an aneurysm. I was shocked, saddened and moved. I wondered if I had done enough. Of course, I can't know if a lifestyle change would have saved his life but I know *it might have* and I'm sure it would of improved the quality of the time he had.

Very few jobs, demands or projects are worth dying for. Even those that risk their lives to protect us do not knowingly put themselves in harms way without being adequately prepared. Many of us, however, continually exhaust our physical and mental healthiness by trying to make everyone else happy.

Countless others I have met express a desire to become fit and healthy, but, "life gets in the way." They are just too busy with work, other obligations, or whatever. But from what I have seen, it is not life that "gets in the way", rather, it is death and debilitating illness. Projects will wait. Appointments can be cancelled. Errands can be rescheduled. You don't have to be on every committee. The kids don't have to play every sport, etc. One man I met quit his personal training program even though his doctor told him it would be bad for his high blood pressure. The man conceded that he made significant progress with his trainer. He had lowered his body fat percentage and blood pressure while increasing his overall fitness and strength. But he felt compelled to quit because a damaging storm had swept through his midwestern town, causing unsightly cracks in the sidewalk around his home. He made the decision to stop training in order to spend six months repairing the cracks in his sidewalk. I don't know if he ever resumed his program. A busy lifestyle with tons of commitments and projects can represent a very real danger as the demands slowly but surely take priority over fitness goals. We may get lots of projects done and fix the material things around the home but the physical home of your body may be developing its own cracks, crevices, and breaking points. Which home do you think really needs the investment of your protection and care? Don't let the urgent crowd out the important.

As a result of my experience with my friend who died, I have become even more straightforward and bold. A week doesn't go by when I don't have a serious conversation with someone about his or her health. Now, when people say that they don't have time because of the kid's schedule, projects at work, demanding jobs, etc. I usually ask the question. "How much time will you have if you're dead, permanently diseased or feeling lousy most of the time?" It doesn't always win me friends but, quite honestly, I don't know what else to say. I have learned to trust in and apply the proverb, "Better are words that sting from a friend, than the kisses of an enemy".

Take time for restoration. Another way to consider it is recreation. Recreation to most of us is golf, fishing, or a day at the beach. Those are in fact excellent ways to re-create. Exercise, however, is also a form of recreation. It actually recreates *and* restores muscle cells and fiber, ligaments, tendons, nerves, arteries, veins, the heart and lungs. At the same time, it refreshes the mind, the emotions, and the spirit. We all need to be dedicated spouses, parents, friends and employees. If we follow the patterns of the wise and successful centenarians, we will be more effective in all we do.

X. Collabor-ation.

> *"Encourage me, and I will not forget you."*
> William Arthur Ward

> *"Excellence encourages one about life generally, it shows the spiritual wealth of the world."*
> T.S. Eliot

> *"The common talk of the struggle for survival has obscured the plain fact that man rose in the world primarily by cooperating, not struggling with his fellows."*
> Herman Muller

Collaboration, according to Webster, means, "to work together". If you are going to be successful in enjoying a lifestyle of fitness and health, you may want to consider building a "team" with which to work. Even though I enjoy working out on my own, I maintain a team of encouraging supporters from whom I learn new ideas, information and motivation.

It is a good idea for you to do the same. In an earlier section of this book, it was noted that those who can train with a good partner have only a 6% dropout rate from a new fitness lifestyle. Those who have no partner end up dropping out at the rate of 43% within the first three months!

Even if you can't find a partner, there are some other ways that you can enhance your likelihood of success. But it is essential that you find someone or *something* to encourage, instruct, and motivate you along the way. The source of this may not be a person whom you can see and talk to each week. It could be a book like this one, or someone you can stay in contact with by phone or e-mail. It is a key principle to success and one we should not ignore.

Speaking of ignoring . . . unfortunately sometimes those around us may be a source of discouragement. In the pursuit of healthiness, we may have to learn to ignore comments intended to weaken our vision of being healthier. Regrettably, change is hard for everyone. When we begin to change, it can put pressure on those around us. They may think they too will have to change in order to deal with your changes. To our surprise and disappointment, even those who love and care about us can discourage us as we attempt to make healthier choices. However, it is important that we "consider the source". Ask yourself, "Is this person really qualified to discourage me in this area"? Unless they have already achieved what it is you want to accomplish, they are *not* qualified to give you sound advice or criticism. In other words, if it were my goal to earn one million dollars per year, I wouldn't strongly consider the advice or criticism of someone who is only making $20,000 a year. The same holds true for a fitness lifestyle.

It is important that we prepare ourselves to deal with the naysayers and dream stealers in our lives that may nitpick away at our vision of a brighter and fitter future. In the book, *Balcony People*, the author describes two types of people we may have in our lives: balcony people and basement people. Balcony people are the ones pulling for us, cheering us on, and encouraging us to succeed. You'll find them in your cheering section, in your balcony. They are treasures, and if you have even one, you are blessed. Basement people, on the other hand, can still be *good people*, but because they may feel threatened or reminded of their own inability to discipline themselves, may knowingly or unknowingly discourage us, drag us down or attempt to hold us back. They can have tremendous influence and may prevent you from succeeding.

Think about the kind of people in your life and then beware of their responses to the changes you make. Seek encouragement from someone or something that builds courage, confidence, and determination. The word, "encourage", in fact, means, "to give courage to". We all need this in our lives. Throughout history, the stories of great achievers tell the tale of difficult challenges being overcome when someone or something came along to provide a shot of courage and confidence.

Consider NBA basketball games. Have you ever noticed how much better the teams play at home versus on the road? Even commentators suggest that the home team has a better chance of winning just because they are playing on their home court. It is simply considered a fact that they will perform better and with more intensity because 17, 000 people will be cheering them. It lifts their spirits and strengthens their resolve because the power of collaboration and encouragement is incredibly strong.

Sometimes, however, the encouragement and confidence building comes from just one player on the team. His leadership, determination and refusal to quit, lifts the spirits of the entire team and they are encouraged to try harder. While most of us cannot expect to have an arena of 17,000 pulling for us with frenetic abandon, we can seek to become the inspirational leader in our own life and pull from a handful of resources to embolden us. The word collaboration begins with the root "coll" as in "to collect". At the back of this book, other valuable books and resources are listed that will give good information, and help keep you on the right path. Find someone or something that will continually tell you that you *can and should* accomplish your goals. Ignore the critics, because, as Teddy Roosevelt said, "it is not the critic who counts, those timid souls who know neither the joy of victory, nor the agony of defeat."

A former employee, whom I will call Lucy, experienced the results of both negative and positive collaboration. Lucy was missing a lot of work when I first met her. Not just a few days, mind you, but a few weeks at a time. When she and I discussed this situation, she would describe all her health problems. It seems that she had chronic pain in her hip and lower back and was told she needed to lose about sixty pounds. As a result of her condition, she required the use of a walker and the extreme pain was contributing to feelings of depression. She would frequently discuss all of the possible surgeries that could be performed and the various medications that were being tried. I asked her if anyone had recommended a fitness routine. I told her of a place where I had worked as a trainer that specialized in helping clients with conditions similar to her own. Many were worker's compensation clients who were being rehabbed back into the workplace. Others were those recovering from heart disease or working to control diabetes and high blood pressure. Many of our clients, I told Lucy, had been helped through a simple weekly workout system.

Upon hearing this, she would always respond, "Well, one of my friends told me about this other doctor . . .". These types of conversation went on for about a year. Eventually it seemed, Lucy ran out of doctors to try. She then turned to chiropractors, herbologists, and acupuncture. While these solutions may have some benefit, I knew in my heart of hearts, that Lucy needed more. However, her circle of influence, her "friends" were all trying to keep Lucy in the circle of sick care. She continued to endure a serenade of illness treating solutions that were *not* getting at the core of her problem, which was an inactive, defeated lifestyle. What Lucy needed was someone who would be honest with her, while teaching her the truth, and encouraging her to realize that she should and could take up a fitness lifestyle. In my position as her boss, I knew I wasn't the one to directly help her.

Eventually, Lucy went out on a worker's compensation claim. She missed a year of work. One day, my boss called me into the office and asked, "Fred, who is this Lucy person?" I explained who she was and asked why he wanted to know. "Did you know that her treatments over the past year have cost $90,000?" he queried? Admittedly, I was not surprised. Having worked in healthcare, I knew that costs climbed quickly. Lucy never did come back to work, opting to retire under her poor health condition.

About one year after that discussion with my boss, I was at the gym one morning. I was busy performing an exercise, when all of a sudden, I hear someone call my name. I looked around but saw no one that I recognized. There was, however, a woman scurrying quickly across the gym floor. "Fred!" she again yelled. I squinted my eyes a little to see if I might recognize this woman. "Fred, it's me, Lucy! "Lucy?" I exclaimed. "Wow, what happened to you?" She did not even look like the same person. My guess is that she had lost over fifty pounds of excess body fat, and added some healthy lean tissue (muscle). She had on a workout outfit, and moved with far more grace and ease than I had ever seen. No longer did she need a walker, slump her shoulders or drag her feet.

Lucy explained, "You know, I met the greatest doctor. He told me that I would never improve until I took control of this myself. He recommended that I hire a trainer and join a gym. He had seen this "prescription" work well for others and he was confident that I could do it and that it could work for me. I guess I listened to too many of the wrong people. I know you tried to tell me the same thing but I had so many others telling me different. I'm so glad I am doing this. I started about nine months ago. I feel so much better. I will never go back to living like that!"

The good news is that Lucy was able to find a physician who saw what she really needed. He was encouraging and upright enough to give it to her straight. Seek out and collaborate with helpful resources. Talk to only those who are walking the walk. Find someone or something to instruct, equip and encourage you. Don't take too seriously anyone who is living less than the best. Misery does indeed love company but that is not the kind of company we want collaborating with us to help us reach a challenging goal. Find an encourager. Follow through on overcoming obstacles and then you will be in position to encourage others in their pursuit of healthiness as well.

XI. Motiv-ation

> *"People often say that motivation doesn't last. Well, neither does bathing—that's why we recommend it daily."*
>
> *Zig Ziglar*

> *"Walking your talk is a great way to motivate yourself. No one likes to live a lie. Be honest with yourself, and you will find the motivation to do what you advise others to do."*
>
> *Vince Poscente*

> *"Desire is the key to motivation, a commitment to excellence— that will enable you to attain the success you seek."*
>
> *Mario Andretti*

Eighty percent of life, according to actor and director Woody Allen, is showing up. That is simple, but profoundly true. The Pareto Principle, also known as the 80/20 rule, does indeed rule in every area of life. The principle, developed in 1906 by Italian economist Vilfredo Pareto, states that 80% of the work is done by 20 % of the people, 80 % of the results come from 20 % of the effort, and so on. We would be wise to use this principle in evaluating our motivation because 80 % of the struggle for most of us who are pursuing healthiness is to *just show up*. Before we get to that though, lets spend a moment looking at this whole subject of motivation.

Motivation, like attitude, is one of those words that have been beaten to a pulp. We've grown a little weary of motivational speakers and rah-rah pep talks. Still, one of the great needs of our society is for people to become motivated. Or is it? Behavior experts tell us that no one really NEEDS more motivation because everyone is already highly motivated. The problem seems to be that many of us don't seem to be motivated towards what is healthy and beneficial to our lives.

The example is often given of the unmotivated, slacker employee, who, when their shift is over, suddenly shifts into high gear and becomes one of the most motivated people in existence. If you were to watch them golfing, gardening or shopping, their entire demeanor and mental attitude are not even close to the person they are at work. Suddenly they may become excited and enthused, displaying energy and passion that is a far cry from the workplace. The same principle often applies in the motivational approach to health and fitness. It seems that many people have a motivational lock on their brains.

There are countless websites and materials that outline, "tips and methods for getting motivated to exercise". Many of these resources do offer helpful and valuable tips for increasing motivation. It is a good idea to read, research and utilize these tips, for exercise, career, relationships and so on.

But preparing to be motivated by reading these resources isn't enough. Sooner or later, the rubber must meet the road. We must cut to the chase and accept that the bottom line to getting and staying motivated is simply getting off our rears and getting in gear. Nike apparently had the answer with their "Just Do it" advertising theme. Or, if you prefer, borrow a line from Larry the Cable Guy and "Get'er done".

The simple formula to "Gettin er done" was something I learned several years ago from an unlikely source. I was working a moonlight job as the coordinator for health promotion in Shasta County, California. It was a grant-funded project that required visiting the homes of senior citizens who were considered "at risk" for health and fitness problems. My assignment was to pay home visits to these folks. I was to assess their nutrition and fitness needs and then determine what might be done to help them maintain their independence.

Frankly, I found this particular experience to be quite depressing. The majority of the people I visited were in shockingly poor shape. They ranged in age from fifty to their late eighties. Many were unable to get around without the use of a walker or wheelchair and were taking up to eight medications. The food on their shelves and in the refrigerators was lacking any real nutritional value. The prognosis for most of these folks looked quite bleak, unless something seriously changed for them. It was quite disheartening as so many of these folks were interesting and endearing.

Perhaps you can imagine how I felt when I received an assignment to visit a gentleman listed as 91 years old. I remember thinking to myself, "Oh, this will be great", envisioning someone barely alive. After a few knocks on the door, a firm voice asked, "whose there?" Finally, a spry looking man, who appeared to be in his mid to late 70's, answered the door. "Yea, what do you want?" he demanded. "I'm here from the *Golden Umbrella* to do a fitness and nutrition assessment," I answered. "What? I don't need any assessment!" he asserted. It was clear to me that he was probably right. Still, I had a job to do. He said, "look Sonny, go see someone else, I'm doing just fine."

In a last ditch effort to get through to this crusty character I said, "Sir, it is clear to me that you are indeed just fine. But maybe you can help some other people. I have spent all week visiting others who are not doing so well and they are all younger than you. Maybe you could share your secret with me. Tell me what you have done to stay in such great shape so that I can share it with others." At that, he smiled. "Secrets! You think there is a secret?" He laughed. "Let me show you my *secret*," he said with a hint of sarcasm. He then invited me into his home and led me down the hallway to what he called his, "get ready room." "This", he said, "is where I get ready for my day." In the room, he had set up a small circuit training gym, complete with a bench, dumbbells, rowing machine and a Nordic track. He began to show me, with enthusiasm, a bit of his routine. His technique and vigor on all of the equipment would have been the envy of people half his age.

"You know, I can't understand why everyone doesn't do this", he said. However, he went on to say that he "doesn't always feel like doing this". He said, "You know, I'm 91 years old. There are many days when I wake up and I feel a bit stiff. But I have learned, if I just come in here and get moving, all of a sudden, I start feeling better, and then, right in the middle of it, I start really enjoying it." He then showed me a poster he had made up and placed on the wall. "Sonny," he said, "this is what you should tell those other people." The poster simply had four short sentences. It said the following:

1) Just show up!
2) Beginning is half done!
3) A body in motion stays in motion.
4) A body in rest, stays at rest.

"I have drilled those words into my head," he said. "In the morning, when I am lying in bed, these words come to mind. It is then that I decide to start moving my body, step by step, into this room. I now know that the way for me to get my exercise done is to just show up in this room. After I show up, I just need to get started. Once I start, I am on my way! I do this everyday now, because I have decided that I am just not ready to rest yet. In fact, you've got to go now, because I have to get to work," he declared. He then informed me that he still works 4 hour a day at a machine shop with his son, "just to keep him in line".

While writing this book over the past year, I have found this "motivational formula" that he shared with me to ring true. In planning to write the book, I spent some time reading and researching, etc. What I found most difficult, however, was simply sitting down and writing. The thought of that seemed daunting. Little thoughts, similar to those that keep some from exercising, started to flood my mind and keep me from writing. Then I came across a book printed in the 1930's on how to write. It said, "Pick up a pen and start writing. As you do, you will make progress. You will make mistakes. Some days will be better than others. Some days will be stinkers, some days everything will flow. You will learn as you go, you will grow as you go. And then, one day, you will hit your stride, and then you will glow with the satisfaction of knowing, you have arrived. At that point, writing will no longer be a struggle or a chore. Rather, it will become a source of pleasure, an inspiration that helps you soar."

With that in mind, I started writing. Dragging myself out of bed at 4:00 am day, after day, after day. Many times I did not feel like it and had almost no idea what I was going to write that day. Fortunately, though, it has happened for me almost precisely as the book predicted. I found that if I just showed up at my desk and began the process of writing, things started gelling. You have read the fruits of my efforts. It is my hope that these fruits have helped motivate you to put forth effort in taking better care of yourself for the rest of your life. The same thing will happen to you, with your workouts, as it happened for me in writing. As you progress in this lifestyle of exercising, eating better, and keeping the vision of an active, fully alive life in mind, you will begin to find great pleasure and satisfaction. But there will be those days, to be sure, when the cobwebs of inactivity seem to be closing in on you. When they hit, and you are struggling with motivation, always remember the words of my 91-year-old friend, "just show up".

XII. Determin-ation.

*"You've got to get up every morning with determination if
you're going to go to bed with satisfaction."*

George Lorimer

*"Life is not a continuum of pleasant choices, but of
inevitable problems that call for strength, **determination**,
and hard work."*

Indian Proverb

*"Mental toughness is many things. It is humility because it
behooves all of us to remember that simplicity is the sign of
greatness and meekness is the sign of true strength. Mental
toughness is spartanism with the qualities of sacrifice, self-
denial, dedication. It is fearlessness, and it is love."*

Vincent Lombardi

One of the consistent themes of life, in virtually all works of good value, is to persevere, to press on, even when it may not make sense to do so. Something good and wonderful seems to happen when we continue striving against all odds. My experience has shown that for millions of people, fitness is a serious, serious, challenge. And though I like to joke a bit, the results of loosing that challenge can be deadly serious. On the other hand, if we can break through, we can enjoy some seriously great results. Winston Churchill, when asked at a high school assembly the key to being successful in life, said that the sum of all the advice he could give boiled down to seven words. Then he slowly but strongly said, "Never, never, never, never, never, never, QUIT!" At that he began to walk off the stage, but then purposefully, he turned and added, "in any endeavor of good purpose or virtue". Taking better care of your self *is* a good purpose and has virtue, not only for your own life, but for others as well. But to start and stay with it for a lifetime, will no doubt require a good dose of determination.

A definition of the word determination that I found on the Internet is, "the act of making up your mind about something." That definition doesn't seem complete. A better definition would include, "with the *firm and final* decision not to give up or quit, despite difficulties, setbacks or obstacles." Determination is a word that can readily be interchanged with the words persistence, tenacity, perseverance, doggedness, endurance, relentlessness, and so on.

Most of us have discovered that anything good in life worth pursuing is going to face inevitable challenges. A pursuit of healthiness will not be an exception. Woodrow Wilson said that persistence alone was omnipotent and ranked it above education, talent, riches, and so on.

I remember learning this from football, in particular, where virtually every other player on my team was more athletic, faster, stronger, and more talented than myself. However, many of the other players did not seem to have as strong a desire or willingness to work hard. I still remember hearing at my very first high school practice, as a skinny awkward freshman, the words of our coach. He stated that, "football, like all of life, was more about desire than anything else. You just have to want it." I remember thinking that was good news, because I knew I did not have a lick of football talent, but I had plenty of desire. When I went to college and tried out for the football team, I remember being shocked at how many far superior players quit during the "dog days" of summer. Some of these players had talent that I could only dream about, and they simply walked away.

As a result, that provided more opportunities and possible playing time for me. By merely doing little more than showing up everyday and applying myself, I was able to succeed beyond anything I had thought possible for myself. The lessons that I learned through my experiences in football reinforced in me tenacity and a commitment to not quit easily or early. I had been fortunate enough to learn that it is *rarely* through talent or special ability that we arrive at the pinnacle of our potential. Instead, it is usually grittiness that can lead us to greater results. In your pursuit of superior health, fitness and wellness, it will ultimately boil down to your ability to keep going that will determine your outcome. As you keep at it, you will make mistakes but you will learn what works best for you. As you stick to your goals, you will begin to experience and enjoy what it feels like to live in a lean, fat-incinerating, anti-aging wellness machine.

It will require a determination that is not commonly found in our culture. But those who develop the determination to train their physical bodies often find it to have an expediential effect. Other areas of life become more manageable and they experience success and victory in unexpected ways.

Determination. Perseverance. Endurance. Our country was born when individuals had these traits as part of their collective mindset. We have grown into greatness because millions of other tough-minded souls worked their hearts out to build a better life, for themselves, and ultimately, for generations to come. Many have given life and limb in their determined efforts to help protect a country that offers everyone a chance to enjoy freedom, life, and the pursuit of *healthiness*. This train of thought has been salt and peppered throughout this book because many of us need more of this "determined" flavoring added to our lives. A zest for living that will not be quenched. We seem to have lost some of this spirit. Indeed, millions of us are being wiped out by killer couches, we have been lulled into a physical lethargy. We have got to get back some of the tenacity of earlier times.

Perhaps like me, you marvel at the hardships endured by previous generations. The difficulties, trying times and heartbreaks they persevered through seem overwhelming. I have been raised in a "soft" culture of comfort and safety. I wonder if I would have had the strength of character, the fiber of fortitude, to persevere, as did my forefathers.

With so many perishing under the perils of poor healthiness, we need a few people to step up to the plate and lead the way back into the "promised land" of awesome health. Will you be among them? Anyone who can still move can make amazing physical improvements. Our bodies are incredible creations that can operate at extremely high levels of performance, if we just give them the chance to do so. It requires ongoing determination to employ just a few simple strategies that are not back breaking. Determine to do this for yourself at first. You will soon enjoy the first fruits of good health, explosive energy and a better appearance. Your determined efforts will produce in you a greater strength of character, a more abundant enthusiasm for life, and an ability to then serve others by encouraging and teaching them to do the same.

Conclusion

"What's it all about, Alfie?"

"And in the end, it's not the years in your life that count. It's the life in your years."

Abraham Lincoln

"What isn't tried won't work"

Jim Sullivan

"In life, as in a football game, hit the line hard"

Theodore Roosevelt

Have you watched a good movie lately? Over the past few years, movies like Lord of the Rings and Gladiator have been big box office hits. Have you noticed that so many of the most popular movies usually involve a struggle? Perhaps the struggle is between good and evil or a struggle to overcome past failures in life. Regardless, we watch as the stars of the show face all kinds of adversity, danger and circumstances that seem hopeless to overcome. Yet, with a relentless desire (and special effects), they press on until they ultimately succeed. You know the ending, the guy gets the girl, the music plays, and then we leave the theatre and go get ice cream. Isn't it interesting that we will spend two to three hours, watching overpaid strangers act out adventures we can usually only imagine being part of. These movies appeal to us, though, because we like to see others overcome insurmountable challenges. It gives us hope and strengthens our resolve to tackle and overcome the challenges we face in our own lives.

In answer to the song, "What's It All About, Alfie?" (From the late 60's), there are a few things that we can say with a degree of certainty and each of them are directly affected by our fitness, health and wellness. The song above was asking questions of the meaning of life. This book, of course, is not meant to answer the meaning of life, although hopefully it will give more meaning to your life. Most of us could use a little more meaning; it helps give our lives purpose and joy. Likewise, it enables us to remain encouraged when times get tough. And life is certainly tough at times. Yes indeed, like it or not, our lives are a "fight to the finish." With that in mind, it only makes sense to make it an adventurous and exciting fight, one in which you and I come out victorious. This is our time, our chance, and our "movie".

It seems that we spend too much time; money and energy watching others live life. Life is not a spectator sport. It is best lived when we are the participants. But we cannot participate nearly as well if we are in poor condition, unprepared to be fully active, or worse yet, diseased. If we are going to live, we might as well make up our minds to live well.

This book was written because it is the passion of my heart to live a fully alive, meaningful, and positively influential life. One of the things I have been blessed with is good health and a love for fitness. Yet, I have worked hard to learn the truth about what health and fitness require. I've worked equally hard to make it work for me by applying what I have learned through physical disciplines. Anything good *is* going to require some work. This is a good thing. Most of us can relate to the innate satisfaction that comes from working hard and seeing the fruit of our labor.

Marketing experts would have you believe otherwise. Whether you are writing a book, selling a product or giving a speech, they will tell you, "make it fast and easy, otherwise they won't buy." Unfortunately, in many cases, that means telling lies. I have chosen to ignore that advice, because if you are like me, you prefer the truth. I believe that many people just want the straightforward, simple truth, along with clear instructions, tools and maybe a little encouragement. I hope that this book has given you that. Most of us have coddled ourselves in comfort to long. Comfort, to a degree, is cool. I like it, you like it, we all scream for it. But, it does not ultimately deliver life on it's own. It must be mixed with short, intentional periods of effort. That effort needs to be effective, consistent and enthusiastic. If we want to enjoy the thrills and spills, the adventure of being and feeling and looking like a lean, fat-incinerating anti-aging machine, it is going to mean leaving the comfort and perceived safety of the couch and getting onto the playing field of a fitness lifestyle.

I hope this book has helped the already knowledgeable, committed and disciplined to pursue their goals with more vigor. But, it is my greatest hope that those who have struggled with motivation, discipline, and perhaps even slothfulness, have been encouraged and equipped to pursue a progressive healthiness lifestyle.

Please contact me via my web site at *www.fitfooddude.com* with questions, suggestions on how I can improve or make this book better, criticisms, or stories of success so that I may continually improve upon this book and encourage others. As I close, I would like to share a story that my wife discovered in the back of a church bulletin. I have shared this at many conferences and always receive several requests for copies. Unfortunately, I am unsure of the author, as all the copies of it we have seen are signed, "anonymous". It is as follows:

The Carpenter

An elderly carpenter was ready to retire. He told his employer contractor of his plans to leave the house building business and live a more leisurely life with his wife, enjoying his extended family. He would miss the paycheck, but he needed to retire. They could get by. The contractor was sorry to see his good worker go and asked if he would build just one more house as a personal favor. The carpenter said yes, but in time it was easy to see that his heart was not in his work. He resorted to shoddy workmanship and used inferior materials. It was an unfortunate way to end a dedicated career.

When the carpenter finished his work, the employer came to inspect the house. He handed the front door key to the carpenter. "This is your house," he said, "my gift to you." The carpenter was shocked! What a shame! If he had only known he was building his own house, he would have done it all so differently.

So it is with us. We build our lives, a day at a time, often putting less than our best into the building. Then with a shock we realize we have to live in the house we have built. If we could do it all over, we'd do it much differently. But we cannot go back. You are the carpenter. Each day you hammer a nail, place a board, and erect a wall. "Life is a do-it-yourself project," someone once said. Your attitudes and the choices you make today, build the "house" you live in tomorrow. Build wisely!

APPENDIX

Speaking Information

For information on scheduling Fred to present a keynote or sessions for your next industry or association conference or employee workshop, please visit his website at *www.fitfooddude.com* or email him at for more information and fee schedules at *fitfooddude@aol.com*

Fred Schafer

Aka (**The Fit Food Dude**)

How to make your next event or convention a hit!! Schedule the Fit Food Dude, who will help make your conference sizzle, impress your socks off, and meet your budget!

Fred Schafer is a keynote speaker and seminar leader specializing in employee wellness, health and fitness. Presenting with enthusiasm and humor, Fred's down to earth style captivates and inspires audiences. His presentations are packed with solid advice and techniques which the participants can implement in their lives immediately to improve their productivity both at work and personally. His vital message has proven not only to entertain and educate all audience members, but to be especially invigorating and life transforming to those who seek immediate and permanent change.

Topics include:

Wellness · Health · Fitness · Confidence · Attitude · Service · Motivation · Lifestyle Management · Self-Discipline · Enthusiasm · Perspective · Goals

"Thank you so much for coming to the ISFSA conference. You were a hit! I really appreciate the message and the time you took to come to Indiana. If you ever need a recommendation I would be glad to add my voice."

Bonnie Burbrink, Indiana

"Fred, thank you so much for coming to our state conference. I can't think of a more perfect speaker for our year. Your thoughts will inspire our Florida team on to better health."

Carol Kehrer, Florida

Further Reading Resources

Strong Women Stay Young by Miriam Nelson
For beginners. Very thorough job of covering the basics for women.
Strong Women Stay Slim by Miriam Nelson
Follow-up to *Strong Women Stay Young*. More info on how strength
   training affects fat metabolism.
Faith Based Fitness by Dr. Kenneth H. Cooper
Medical program that uses spiritual motivation to achieve
   maximum health and add years to your life
Stretching by Gary Anderson
Excellent guide to flexibility/stretching
Getting Stronger by Bill Pearl
Sport specific training programs
Holy Sweat by Tim Hansel
Character Qualities to Take Us higher
Living Longer Stronger by Ellington Darden
Good starter book for men.
Strength Training Past Fifty by Wayne Westcott Ph.D.
One of the Country's best authorities on strength training benefits
   for seniors.
Lift Weights to Lose Weight by Kathy Smith
Famous aerobics star has discovered the power of resistance training!!

Strength & Power for Young Athletes by A. Faigenbaum and Wayne Westcott

All people are considered athletes!! The principles are the same for young males and females.

Biomarkers: The 10 Keys to Prolonging Vitality by William Evans, Ph. D.

Hint. The primary message of the book is to add muscle to your body!

The Schwarzbein Principle by Diana Schwarzbein, M.D.

Excellent nutrition guide. Details myths on cholesterol, diabetes, etc

Neanderthin (Eat like a caveperson for a lean strong body)by Ray Audette

I do not agree with everything in this book, but the concept makes sense, and is interesting.

General References

Introduction

Does the food pyramid need revision? (2003, July) *Fitness Management*. 21.

Carrol, J. (2002, June). Attack on the food pyramid. CCCCC Food Program.

Chapter 1

American's health priorities not in line with practices. (2001, May). *Fitness Management*. 8.

The Secret of Long Life (2001, December). *Modern Maturity*. 44(6), 13.

Evans, W. (1992) *Biomarkers: The 10 keys to Vitality*. Fireside.

Lovallo, W. (1997). *Stress & Health* London: SAGE Publications, Ltd.

Schwarzenegger, Arnold (1985) *Encyclopedia of Modern Body Building* New York: Simon & Schuster

Chapter 4

Hatfield, F. (1996) Fitness: *The Complete Guide*. Santa Barbara, California: ISSA

Chapter 7

Arria, S. (2003, July). Is it really health care? (On-line). http://
www.issaonline.com/e-fitwire/issue6/index.cfm

Billions of dollars, thousands of lives. (2001, November). (On-Line). www.agingresearch.org

Chapter 9

Westcott, W. (2002, December). Strength training for the aging adult. (Online). www.fitnessworld.com/info/info_pages/library/strength/strength695.html

Todd, T., & Todd, J. (1985) *Lift your Way to Youthful Fitness.* Boston: Little, Brown

Connelly, A.S. (2001) *Body RX.* New York: G.P. Putnam's Sons.

Kaplan, P. (1996) *Transform!* Fort Lauderdale, Florida: Great Atlantic Publishing Group.

Chapter 10

Brehm, B. (2000, March). Successful weight control: help clients redefine success. *Fitness Management.* 32-34.

Chapter 11

Nelson, M.E. (2000) *Strong Women Stay Young.* New York: Bantam Books.

Hahn, F., & Eades, M. (2003) *The Slow Burn Fitness Revolution.* New York: Broadway Books.

Willix, R. (1994) *You Can Feel Good All The Time.* Baltimore, MD: Health for Life

Study shows link between exercise type, intensity and chd. (2002, December). *Recreational Sports & Fitness.* 29-30.

Krucoff, C. (2000, Sept./Oct. 2000). Weight training for your heart. *The Saturday Evening Post.* 26-27.

Duschinski, T. (1994, Sept./Oct.). Benefits of Weight Training. *New Man.* 78-79.

Infanti, S. (2001, July). Resistance training is residual. *Record Searchlight.* D-3.

Pumping iron could aid in cancer fight. (2003, October). *Record Searchlight* (AP).

Johnstone, B. (2003). Exercise Science: Theory & Practice. Sudbury, ON Canada:BODYworx

Colgan, M., & Weider, B. Bodybuilding For A Heart. Quebec, Canada: IFFB

Strength Training and Aging (1999). Keiser Institute On Aging. Fresno, Ca: Keiser Corporation

Chapter 12

Yoga injuries on the rise. (2003, February). *Club Industy*. 8.

How much is too much? Reebok Alliance newsletter. 33-34. *www.reebokalliance.com*

Chapter 13

Yessis, M. (2003, November). Using free weights for stability training. *Fitness Management.* 19(12), 26-28.

Westcott, W. (2003, December). The learning curve for women's weight-loss programs. Fitness Management. 19(13), 38-41.

Sichel, H. (2004, February). Power Pilates. *Personal Fitness Professional.* 29-30.

Chapter 14

Claps, F. (2002, December). Fibromyalgia:exercise can offer relief for people who live with this painful malady. *Muscle & Fitness/Hers.*

Kraemer, W., & Fleck, S. (1993) *Strength Training For Young Athletes.* Champaign, IL: Human Kinetics

McAlpine, K. Little lifters. *Spirit Magazine*

Chapter 16

Pofeldt, E. (June, 2003). The battle of the diet docs. *Fortune Small Business.* 56.

Hall, B. R.D. (2001, November). Time to eat. *Muscle Media.* 89-90.

Brehm, B. (2001, July). The Paleolithic lifestyle: helping stone age bodies adapt to modern times. *Fitness Management.* 30.

Chapter 17

Schwarzbein, D.(1999) The Schwarzbein Factor. Deerfield Beach, FL: health Communications, Inc.

Chapter 18

Pofeldt, E. (June, 2003). The battle of the diet docs. *Fortune Small Business*. 56.

Chapter 20

McGinnis, A. L. (1990) *The Power of Optimism*. Harper Collins.

Taylor, S. E. (1995). *Health Psychology*. New York: McGraw-Hill, Inc.

Smid, J. (2000, February). Smile-it'll make you live longer. (On-line). *www.exn.ca*

Brehm, B. (2002, May). Using the power of imagination to plan for behavior-change success. Fitness Management. 27.

Kaplan, P. (1999, July/August). How do you motivate clients? *Personal Fitness Professional*. 18-21.

Satcher, D. (2000, March). The physical approach to better mental health. *Club Business International*. 120-123.

Related Websites and Resources

Exercise Instruction

- www.exrx.net
- www.strength training.asimba.com
- www.orthodox.net/link

Nutrition Information

- www.wheyoflife.org
- www.glycemicindex.com

Personal Trainer Locator and Qualification Guidelines

- www.ideafit.com

Dumbbells and Ankle Weights

- www.powerblock.com
- www.probell.com
- www.nefitco.com/ankle_weight_20lb.html

Body Fat Calipers and Measuring Tapes

- www.accufitness.com.

About the Author

Fred Schafer, founder and director of "Fit Food Dude Enterprises", is a Certified Fitness Trainer with a 30-year background in the fitness, health and wellness field. In 1995, he established a personal fitness training service after observing so many people fail in their sincere efforts to achieve their health and fitness goals. He began to teach others the true principles of fitness and nutrition which prevented them from falling victim to the slick marketing of infomercials, fitness fraud, and nutritional nonsense that we are bombarded with daily.

Fred knew that people could reach their goals if they followed the steps he had identified for successful physical transformation. For a number of years he worked part-time with others one on one, while working full-time as a Director of Food/Nutrition for several school districts. Over the past few years, he has moved to conducting health, fitness and wellness seminars for conferences and organizations, as this allows him to impact a greater number of people in less time.

He continues to work as a Food/Nutrition Director, is married with three children. He has a proven track record of outstanding success as a fitness trainer, motivational speaker, school district administrator, research scientist, author, marketing consultant, and health care manager and in management within the hotel and restaurant industry. Fred can relate to the busy lives of others while helping them to be successful in enjoying a lifetime of extraordinary fitness, health, and wellness.

Credentials

ISSA Certified Personal Fitness Trainer
Past Director of Nutrition Services, Redding Specialty Hospital
Present Director of Food/Nutrition for Two School Districts
California Dept. of Education Advisory Vice Chairperson Student Nutrition
Josephine Morris Student Nutrition Scholarship Recipient
Previous Coordinator for Shasta County Health Promotion Project
B.S. in Food and Nutrition, Indiana University of Pennsylvania
M.S. in Wellness Promotion

Edwards Brothers Malloy
Thorofare, NJ USA
May 19, 2013